Managing Complications in Paediatric Anaesthesia

Managing Complications in Paediatric Anaesthesia

Martin Jöhr

Department of Anaesthesia, Luzerner Kantonsspital, Lucerne, Switzerland

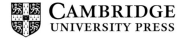

CAMBRIDGE
UNIVERSITY PRESS

University Printing House, Cambridge CB2 8BS, United Kingdom

One Liberty Plaza, 20th Floor, New York, NY 10006, USA

477 Williamstown Road, Port Melbourne, VIC 3207, Australia

314–321, 3rd Floor, Plot 3, Splendor Forum, Jasola District Centre, New Delhi – 110025, India

79 Anson Road, #06–04/06, Singapore 079906

Cambridge University Press is part of the University of Cambridge.

It furthers the University's mission by disseminating knowledge in the pursuit of education, learning, and research at the highest international levels of excellence.

www.cambridge.org
Information on this title: www.cambridge.org/9781316629109
DOI: 10.1017/9781316823064

© Martin Jöhr 2018

First published 2018

Printed and bound in Great Britain by Clays Ltd, Elcograph S.p.A.

A catalogue record for this publication is available from the British Library

Library of Congress Cataloging-in-Publication Data
Names: Johr, Martin, author.
Title: Managing complications in paediatric anaesthesia / Martin Johr.
Description: New York, NY : Cambridge University Press, 2018. |
    Includes bibliographical references and index.
Identifiers: LCCN 2018012433 | ISBN 9781316629109 (pbk. : alk. paper)
Subjects: | MESH: Anesthesia–adverse effects | Intraoperative
    Complications | Child | Infant | Case Reports
Classification: LCC RD139 | NLM WO 440 | DDC 617.9/6083–dc23
    LC record available at https://lccn.loc.gov/2018012433

ISBN 978-1-316-62910-9 Paperback

....

To the parents of our young patients, who frequently have to cope with uncertainty and suffering, and sometimes even with grief

Contents

Acknowledgements

I wish to thank Dr Felix Hess, Dr Roland Jundt and Professor Gregor Schubiger for their teaching and guidance on my way towards a career in paediatric anaesthesiology. I am also very grateful for the exchange of ideas, the support and friendship I experienced with Professor Isabelle Murat and Professor Bernard Dalens.

Special thanks go to Professor Thomas M. Berger for our inspiring daily discussions, and for his inestimable help in editing the first draft of this book.

My wife Benedikta deserves the most heartfelt acknowledgement; without her never-ending patience and support throughout my adult life I would not have been privileged to enjoy a rich professional career, and many projects, such as writing this book, would never have been accomplished.

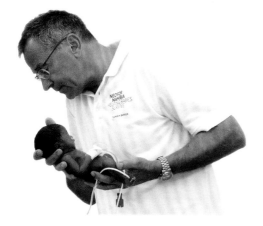

Professor Thomas M. Berger helping babies survive on a mission in Africa.

Abbreviations

ADARPEF	Association des Anesthésistes Réanimateurs Pédiatriques d'Expression Française (the French-language society of paediatric anaesthesia)
ADHD	attention deficit hyperactivity disorder
ASD	autism spectrum disorder
ASIS	anterior superior iliac spine
BChE	butyrylcholinesterase, formerly pseudocholinesterase
BIPAP	bilevel inspiratory positive airway pressure
BIS	bispectral index
CAS	central anticholinergic syndrome
CDH	congenital diaphragmatic hernia
CK	creatine kinase
CMT	Charcot–Marie–Tooth disease
CNS	central nervous system
CPAP	continuous positive airway pressure
CRP	C-reactive protein
CSF	cerebrospinal fluid
CT	computed tomography
ECG	electrocardiogram
ECMO	extracorporeal membrane oxygenation
EEG	electroencephalogram
EMLA	eutectic mixture of local anaesthetics
ENT	ear nose and throat (surgery)
ETT	endotracheal tube
EXIT	ex utero intrapartum treatment
FiO$_2$	fraction of inspired oxygen
GCS	Glasgow Coma Scale
HbA$_{1C}$	glycated haemoglobin
HFOV	high-frequency oscillatory ventilation
ICU	intensive care unit
IVC	inferior vena cava
LMA	laryngeal mask airway
LED	light-emitting diode (light source)
MAC	minimal alveolar concentration
Met-Hb	methaemoglobin
MH	malignant hyperthermia
MRI	magnetic resonance imaging
NADPH	nicotinamide adenine dinucleotide phosphate
NIBP	non-invasive blood pressure
NICU	neonatal intensive care unit
NSAID	non-steroidal anti-inflammatory drug
OR	operating room
PCA	patient-controlled analgesia
pCO$_2$	partial pressure of carbon dioxide
PEEP	positive end-expiratory pressure
PICC	peripherally inserted central catheter
PICU	paediatric intensive care unit
PLSVC	persistent left superior vena cava
PRIS	propofol infusion syndrome
PTC	post-tetanic count
RAE	Ring–Adair–Elwyn
RSV	respiratory syncytium virus

RYR1	ryanodine-1 receptor
SCFE	slipped capital femoral epiphysis
SIADH	syndrome of inadequate secretion of antidiuretic hormone
SVC	superior vena cava
TAP	transverse abdominal plane
TCI	target-controlled infusion
TIVA	total intravenous anaesthesia
TOF	train-of-four
UAC	umbilical arterial catheter
UK	United Kingdom
URTI	upper respiratory tract infection

1 Introduction

'When things go wrong in paediatric anaesthesia' was the working title of this book. Despite his conviction that every anaesthetic should be performed as perfectly as possible, during his professional career the author has observed numerous patients in whom the clinical course was suboptimal, and even some in whom it resulted in harm. In the majority of these cases, at least at some time point, a different clinical decision or an alternative action would have completely changed the outcome.

Based on case presentations, this book aims to give advice on how to avoid some of the most common clinical pitfalls, and to enable anaesthetists to provide safe care to our small patients, following the motto of Albert Einstein, 'A clever person solves a problem, a wise person avoids it.'

The author has spent over 40 years in clinical medicine, training in a university hospital and in several district hospitals. Ultimately, he was responsible for the section of paediatric anaesthesia in a major teaching hospital in Switzerland. The most inspiring time in his professional life was an 18-year period he spent with Professor Thomas M. Berger, a paediatrician, a gifted neonatologist and a great teacher. In many situations, this strong collaboration between an anaesthetist and a paediatrician/neonatologist enabled the author to reach a clear view of the best course of action and to come to conclusions that hopefully are relevant in helping others to learn.

Some of the adverse events described occurred many decades ago, and only fragments of the story could be remembered. In the more recent cases, where more detail is provided, every effort was made to track down the patient and to ask for permission from patient and/or parents to include the individual history in this book. The author is inestimably grateful to all of them for their support in improving the perioperative care of future generations of children.

2 Concepts and Strategy

General Safety Rules: Identification of the Patient and the Type of Surgery

Case

Many decades ago, a 6-year-old boy was scheduled for the removal of pins from his right elbow. After inhalational induction, the airway was secured with a laryngeal mask airway (LMA). The child was allowed to breathe spontaneously, an NSAID was given and wound infiltration by the surgeon was planned.

After skin disinfection and draping, surgery started on the right elbow, where a scar was clearly visible. In the meantime, the anaesthesia team filled out the protocol, and realized that, in contrast to the surgical list, the anaesthetist had written 'pin removal left elbow' at the preoperative visit. The senior anaesthetist advised the trainee to correct the protocol, because, as a general rule, the surgical list was assumed to provide the correct facts. However, despite surgical exploration down to the bone, no pins could be seen or palpated, and the surgeon requested to see the x-ray. This x-ray revealed that the reduction and fixation of the fracture had been performed on the left elbow. Obviously, the indication of the site on the surgical list was wrong. Surgery proceeded on the opposite side, and the parents were informed about the error.

Discussion

This case of **wrong-site surgery** illustrates the importance of high-quality team performance. At first glance, wrong-site surgery seems to be a surgical problem. However, in this case, the anaesthesia team could have intervened and therefore has to share the blame. Whenever the slightest discrepancies are noted, alarm bells should ring and the situation has to be re-evaluated. This was not done in this case.

In those days, no use was made of a **patient identification** bracelet, or a formal checklist, or marking of the operation site. None of these was thought to be necessary. Patient identification is of paramount importance. The author is aware of a situation in which rectal premedication with midazolam 15 mg was given to the 3-month-old baby on the arm of the nanny and not to the 5-year-old patient playing hidden in a corner of the room. The children's nanny had a sociocultural background that would not allow her to object to decisions of medical personnel. The author was impressed by this event and subsequently insisted, against the traditional attitude in his institution, that an identification bracelet must be introduced.

The use of a simple **surgical checklist** before skin incision, a so-called 'time-out', would have prevented this event without any doubt. Checklists are a strategy to improve patient safety and perioperative care (Treadwell *et al.* 2014). The introduction of a surgical safety checklist has even been shown to reduce hospital mortality (van Klei *et al.* 2012). If the

(a)

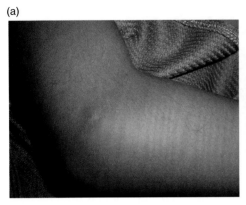

(b)

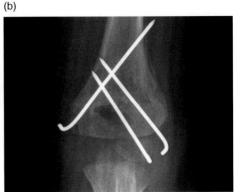

Figure 2.1a Right elbow with a scar following a mosquito bite.

Figure 2.1b X-ray of left elbow with pins. In this more recent case, surgery was performed on the correct site.

baseline quality of the perioperative process is high, however, the additional impact of a checklist may be small, and it may not necessarily further improve outcome. This has been shown in adult (Urbach *et al.* 2014) and in paediatric populations (O'Leary *et al.* 2016). The delicious irony of the study findings is that, since the mean outcome remained unchanged, there must have been improvement in some institutions, whereas in others the implementation of a checklist in a formerly perfectly functioning system worsened outcome. With this in mind, it is probably good to concentrate on a few, really important checklists (Grigg 2015). The author believes that an inundation with checklists (especially with those in which electronic checkboxes are ticked on a screen) will not necessarily contribute to improvement of safety (de Vries *et al.* 2009).

Almost a decade ago, the author began to work through a very simple oral **checklist before the induction of anaesthesia**: patient, intervention, absent allergies, drawn-up medications (hypnotic, relaxant and atropine), anaesthesia machine with tubing, and airway equipment (laryngoscope with the correct blade and the correctly sized tube). This improved safety, because in numerous cases something could be added or improved.

Finally, it is always smart to have a look at the site of surgery before surgery starts. In the presented case, the anaesthetist would not have palpated any pins. This would have been unusual after an elbow fracture and, consequently, the x-ray would have been checked. In addition, such an evaluation might also allow some prediction of the potential duration of surgery.

Summary and Recommendations

This case of wrong-site surgery emphasizes the importance of a high-quality, standardized process in perioperative care.

Following a preoperative checklist (so-called 'time-out') would surely have prevented this complication.

Wrong-site surgery is not a complication caused exclusively by the surgeon. In most cases, it is the consequence of insufficient team performance. In the presented case, the anaesthesia team noted the discrepancy but, unfortunately, none of the members spoke up to stop the start of surgery.

References

de Vries, E.N., Hollmann, M.W., Smorenburg, S.M., *et al.* (2009). Development and validation of the SURgical PAtient Safety System (SURPASS) checklist. *Qual Saf Health Care*, 18, 121–126.

Grigg, E. (2015). Smarter clinical checklists: how to minimize checklist fatigue and maximize clinician performance. *Anesth Analg*, 121, 570–573.

O'Leary, J.D., Wijeysundera, D.N., & Crawford, M.W. (2016). Effect of surgical safety checklists on pediatric surgical complications in Ontario. *CMAJ*, 188, E191–E198.

Treadwell, J.R., Lucas, S., & Tsou, A.Y. (2014). Surgical checklists: a systematic review of impacts and implementation. *BMJ Qual Saf*, 23, 299–318.

Urbach, D.R., Govindarajan, A., Saskin, R., *et al.* (2014). Introduction of surgical safety checklists in Ontario, Canada. *N Engl J Med*, 370, 1029–1038.

van Klei, W.A., Hoff, R.G., van Aarnhem, E.E., *et al.* (2012). Effects of the introduction of the WHO 'Surgical Safety Checklist' on in-hospital mortality: a cohort study. *Ann Surg*, 255, 44–49.

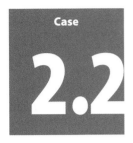

Adequate Anaesthetic Plan

Case

Many decades ago, an 8-month-old boy, weighing 8 kg, presented with a rapidly growing cavernous haemangioma involving the neck and face on the right side. The surgical plan was to ligate the external carotid artery, and then, if feasible, partially resect the haemangioma. Both a low platelet count, 20 000/μl, and an elevated prothrombin time were known preoperatively.

A moderately experienced anaesthesiology trainee was in charge, intermittently supervised by a senior staff member. Anaesthesia was induced with ketamine and succinylcholine; enflurane and repeated boluses of ketamine and alcuronium (a non-depolarizing muscle relaxant with some potential for histamine release) were used for maintenance. Monitoring included a precordial stethoscope, ECG and the new oscillometric blood pressure monitoring device Dinamap. The described incident happened well before the introduction of pulse oximetry into clinical practice, continuous capnography was not yet available, and invasive blood pressure monitoring had never been used in children in this institution before.

First, venous access was achieved by surgical cut-down at both elbows, and two units of platelets (about 70 ml each) were administered. Shortly after incision at the neck, the Dinamap could not record 'interpretable values' and was thought to be malfunctioning. Noise impeded the use of the precordial stethoscope. Only minutes later, the surgeon could no longer feel the pulsating carotid artery used for orientation. This was followed by bradycardia with wide complexes on the ECG screen.

The supervising anaesthetist rushed in and suggested the administration of Lanoxin, a digitalis preparation, and left to calculate the dose. The trainee remembered that he had used dopamine in adults in cases with cardiovascular instability and started a dopamine drip. Surgery was cancelled, and the infant was transferred to the ICU. Despite the fact that circulation could be restored, the pupils remained dilated and the patient died.

Discussion

This case highlights the importance of an **adequate anaesthetic plan** and the understanding of the pathophysiology of the underlying disease. The anaesthesia team was not aware of congestive heart failure caused by massive hypercirculation through large haemangioma vessels (Fig. 2.2). Fluid overload by approximately 20 ml/kg of platelet concentrates led to circulatory collapse in this frail patient. Today, hyperdynamic pump failure would be documented by echocardiography prior to surgery and would therefore be known to the anaesthetist. Undoubtedly, such a complex case would be done by a senior staff member and not by a superficially supervised young trainee. It is well known that the experience of

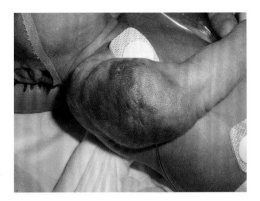

Figure 2.2 Another large haemangioma related to increased cardiac output. A photo of the boy from the presented case is unfortunately not available.

the anaesthetist and the age of the patient are the main predictors of complications (Habre *et al.* 2017).

From today's point of view, **invasive monitoring**, including an arterial line, would be considered standard for such a case. In addition, vasoactive drug drips, e.g. dopamine or noradrenaline, would be prepared before starting the case. In those days, oscillometric blood pressure monitoring was a new technology, and invasive blood pressure monitoring, both in adults and in children, was mainly used in cardiac centres. In this institution, it had never before been used in children. At the time, many practitioners felt that arterial and central venous lines could not be used in small children. Physicians working in university centres, except perhaps for those with experience in dedicated cardiac units, shared this attitude. Surgical cut-downs were often performed for the insertion of venous lines. Pulse oximetry did not yet exist, and capnography was not available.

In summary, from today's perspective, a team with insufficient experience started the case without being adequately equipped and prepared. This case impressively shows that the customary standard in an institution does not necessarily meet the desirable standard. This emphasizes the importance of continuous exchange between institutions. What was standard practice yesterday may no longer be acceptable today.

Kasabach–Merrit syndrome is characterized by giant haemangioma(s) and thrombocytopenia, often complicated by hyperdynamic cardiac failure (Kumar *et al.* 2013, Wang *et al.* 2014). Recently, beta-blockers, especially propranolol, have become the first-line treatment for cutaneous (Kum & Khan 2014) as well as subglottic (Hardison *et al.* 2016) haemangiomas. For these conditions, treatment with surgical excision or laser therapy has become rare. Initially, the patient should be monitored, since hypotension, bradycardia and hypoglycaemia can occur. Obviously, beta-blockers should not be used in patients with high-output cardiac failure.

Summary and Recommendations

The presented case illustrates that an insufficiently prepared and equipped team can contribute to a bad outcome. To be fair, the described events should be seen in their historical context, when the approach taken was the accepted standard of care.

Another important conclusion that can be drawn from this case is the fact that when blood pressure cannot be measured, it is usually not a technical problem, but blood pressure is really low and urgent treatment is needed.

The key message of this case is that every anaesthetist should continuously examine his or her own practice. Improvements in the field of anaesthesiology will continue to be made. What was standard practice yesterday may no longer be good enough today.

References

Habre, W., Disma, N., Virag, K., *et al.* (2017). Incidence of severe critical events in paediatric anaesthesia (APRICOT): a prospective multicentre observational study in 261 hospitals in Europe. *Lancet Respir Med*, 5, 412–425.

Hardison, S., Wan, W., & Dodson, K.M. (2016). The use of propranolol in the treatment of subglottic hemangiomas: a literature review and meta-analysis. *Int J Pediatr Otorhinolaryngol*, 90, 175–180.

Kum, J.J. & Khan, Z.A. (2014). Mechanisms of propranolol action in infantile hemangioma. *Dermatoendocrinol*, 6, e979699.

Kumar, S., Taneja, B., Saxena, K.N., *et al.* (2013). Anaesthetic management of a neonate with Kasabach–Merritt syndrome. *Indian J Anaesth*, 57, 292–294.

Wang, P., Zhou, W., Tao, L., *et al.* (2014). Clinical analysis of Kasabach–Merritt syndrome in 17 neonates. *BMC Pediatr*, 14, 146.

Case

2.3

Understanding the Surgical Procedure and the Patient's Physiology

Case

A 7-month-old boy, weighing 6 kg, with Cornelia de Lange syndrome was scheduled for laparoscopic fundoplication and gastrostomy tube insertion. He had a cleft palate. Echocardiographic findings were normal with the exception of an aberrant right subclavian artery (so-called arteria lusoria).

From previous anaesthetics, difficult intubation was anticipated. He was induced by mask and fibreoptically intubated via the Frei endoscopy mask with a size 3.0 cuffed endotracheal tube (ETT). Anaesthesia was maintained over more than 6 hours with sevoflurane 2 V%, small doses of fentanyl, and mivacurium as a continuous infusion. A 4F double-lumen central venous catheter was inserted into the right internal jugular vein. A 2F 5 cm arterial line was inserted under ultrasound guidance into the right radial artery without difficulties and a stable tracing was observed.

When the surgeons were working on the fundoplication and requested the insertion of a large-bore orogastric tube, the arterial tracing suddenly disappeared. A similar episode occurred during gastroscopy, which was performed for gastrostomy tube insertion (Fig. 2.3). When repeated flushing of the right radial line was unsuccessful, oscillometric blood pressure measurements on the left arm were obtained. Patient positioning was carefully checked to rule out the possibility that direct pressure on the right arm was responsible for the loss of the arterial tracing. It was then speculated that the flat arterial tracing could have something to do with the use of a large gastric tube in the presence of the arteria lusoria.

When fundoplication was completed, the gastric tube was removed, and immediately a normal arterial tracing reappeared. Because a gastrostomy tube was also inserted, there was no need for another gastric tube.

Discussion

This case of compression of an aberrant subclavian artery by a large gastric tube and then by a gastroscope illustrates that surgical manipulations can interfere unexpectedly with anaesthesia management. It also shows that every small detail, such as the presence of an arteria lusoria, should be evaluated preoperatively for its potential relevance to the intraoperative course.

The most common abnormality of the aortic arch (0.6–1.4%) is an aberrant right subclavian artery, a so-called **arteria lusoria** (Polguj *et al.* 2014). The vessel arises from the descending aorta and runs behind the oesophagus and the trachea to the right clavicular region. While the large majority of patients are asymptomatic, compression of adjacent

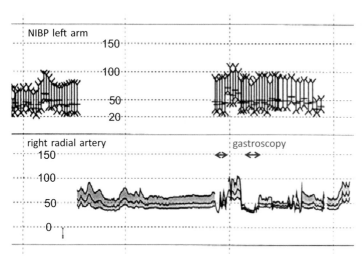

Figure 2.3 The disappearance of the arterial tracing during the insertion of a large gastric tube or a gastroscope in a child with an arteria lusoria.

structures can cause symptoms. Compression of the oesophagus can cause dysphagia (Barone *et al.* 2016) and compression of the trachea can cause dyspnoea and stridor (Derbel *et al.* 2012). Interestingly, as demonstrated by the presented case, a large foreign body in the oesophagus can compress the subclavian artery, leading to the disappearance of the pulse at the wrist. This phenomenon has already been reported during transoesophageal echocardiography in a neonate (Koinig *et al.* 2003). If unknown, the presence of an arteria lusoria presents a major risk during oesophageal surgery (Lacout *et al.* 2012). The author is aware of a baby with oesophageal atresia where this large abnormal arterial vessel lying behind the oesophagus was not correctly identified and ligated. Immediately, the pulse oximeter signal from the right hand was lost. An arteria lusoria may also be detected during right transradial coronary interventions (Allen *et al.* 2016). Associated vascular malformations may include a common carotid trunk or a left-sided vena cava.

Cornelia de Lange syndrome is a clinically variable disorder that affects multiple organs (Boyle *et al.* 2015). Severe intellectual disability and a difficult airway due to a short neck and micrognathia are major challenges for the paediatric anaesthetist. But, in contrast to current belief, there is no elevated risk for malignant hyperthermia (Emerson & Nguyen 2017).

Summary and Recommendations

The presented case of a child with an arteria lusoria interfering with blood pressure monitoring when a large gastric tube was in place shows that even after a careful preoperative workup, the anaesthetist may fail to recognize the cause of the observed changes. Only lifelong experience and learning will further improve competence.

This story also supports the practice of always installing oscillometric blood pressure monitoring equipment on a different extremity when an arterial line is used, in order to have a valuable back-up ready when the invasive method fails.

References

Allen, D., Bews, H., Vo, M., *et al.* (2016). Arteria lusoria: an anomalous finding during right transradial coronary intervention. *Case Rep Cardiol*, 2016, 8079856.

Barone, C., Carucci, N.S., & Romano, C. (2016). A rare case of esophageal dysphagia in children: aberrant right subclavian artery. *Case Rep Pediatr*, 2016, 2539374.

Boyle, M.I., Jespersgaard, C., Brondum-Nielsen, K., *et al.* (2015). Cornelia de Lange syndrome. *Clin Genet*, 88, 1–12.

Derbel, B., Saaidi, A., Kasraoui, R., *et al.* (2012). Aberrant right subclavian artery or arteria lusoria: a rare cause of dyspnea in children. *Ann Vasc Surg*, 26, 419.e1–4.

Emerson, B. & Nguyen, T. (2017). Are children with Cornelia de Lange syndrome at risk for malignant hyperthermia? *Paediatr Anaesth*, 27, 215–216.

Koinig, H., Schlemmer, M., & Keznickl, F.P. (2003). Occlusion of the right subclavian artery after insertion of a transoesophageal echocardiography probe in a neonate. *Paediatr Anaesth*, 13, 617–619.

Lacout, A., Khalil, A., Figl, A., *et al.* (2012). Vertebral arteria lusoria: a life-threatening condition for oesophageal surgery. *Surg Radiol Anat*, 34, 381–383.

Polguj, M., Chrzanowski, L., Kasprzak, J.D., *et al.* (2014). The aberrant right subclavian artery (arteria lusoria): the morphological and clinical aspects of one of the most important variations: a systematic study of 141 reports. *ScientificWorldJournal*, 2014, 292734.

Organization and Fasting Times

Case

A long time ago, a 5-month-old girl with trigonocephaly was scheduled for frontal cranioplasty. To allow sufficient time for preoperative preparation, surgery was scheduled for 09:30 am, following another, shorter case in this operating room. At this institution, nurses traditionally used the time indicated on the surgical list to determine the beginning of the preoperative fasting period. Consequently, the fasting period for the patient started at 05:30 am.

The anaesthetic plan included general endotracheal anaesthesia, an arterial line, central venous access and the insertion of a bladder catheter. To allow sufficient time for a younger colleague to perform these interventions in a training setting, the child was ordered to theatre at 07:30 am, 2 hours before the intended start of surgery.

Anaesthesia was induced by mask with halothane and nitrous oxide. Peripheral venous access was obtained and atracurium was injected. Ventilation by mask was uneventful, but intubation with a size 4.0 uncuffed RAE tube was difficult and ended up with oesophageal intubation. Trial ventilation immediately led to inflation of the stomach, and its milky content completely filled the mouth up to the lips. The mouth was suctioned and the endotracheal tube (ETT) was removed. When mask ventilation was attempted, there was further regurgitation of milk into the mouth. Finally, intubation was successful, the stomach was emptied and relevant volumes of a milky fluid were suctioned from the trachea. Unfortunately, ventilation remained difficult with an FiO_2 requirement of 80% to maintain oxygen saturations above 90%.

Surgery was cancelled and the girl was transferred to the intensive care unit, where she was successfully weaned and extubated 6 hours later. When the case was reviewed, it was discovered that the infant had been fed 200 ml of formula milk two hours before induction of anaesthesia.

Discussion

The presented case of massive milk aspiration leading to severely impaired gas exchange and cancellation of surgery illustrates the importance of a well-structured perioperative process. While the local rule to fast infants according to the scheduled beginning of surgery works perfectly well for routine cases, when induction takes 10–20 minutes, it may cause a problem when induction takes almost 2 hours and the child is ordered to theatre much earlier. In this particular situation the nurses should have been instructed to give the last meal earlier, to guarantee an adequate time interval between the last meal and anaesthesia induction.

Fasting guidelines were introduced to reduce the risk of pulmonary aspiration. Most commonly the 2–4–6-hour rule is followed: 2 hours for clear fluids, 4 hours for breast milk and 6 hours for formula milk and solid food. These guidelines are based on expert opinion, and there is at least some consensus in North America (American Society of Anesthesiology 2017) and throughout Europe (Smith *et al.* 2011). However, slight local variations exist. The Scandinavian guidelines do not distinguish between breast milk and formula, but instead use an age limit for milk: under 6 months, 4 hours; over 6 months, 6 hours (Soreide *et al.* 2005). The German guidelines are the most liberal, quoting 4 hours for milk during the first year of life (Becke *et al.* 2007).

The type of milk does markedly influence the speed of gastric emptying; it is faster after human breast milk, compared to whey-predominant, casein-predominant formula preparations or even cow's milk (Billeaud *et al.* 1990). Cow's milk should be handled like solid food. On the other hand, in a case of aspiration, both human breast milk and formula milk can cause severe disturbances of gas exchange (O'Hare *et al.* 1996). Throughout his professional career, the author has followed the Scandinavian guidelines, allowing infants younger than 6 months to be fed up to 4 hours before surgery, since a 6-hour fasting period for a 2-week-old neonate with a mother who cannot breastfeed would be far too long.

Today, the focus has shifted, recognizing the importance of **sufficient hydration** and good patient comfort before surgery. Traditionally, the fasting period for most patients has been far too long (Engelhardt *et al.* 2011). This has been shown to lead to ketone body formation and has been associated with haemodynamic instability following induction (Dennhardt *et al.* 2016). Today, there is consensus that infants and small children should drink until 2 hours before surgery; but, in a busy clinical surrounding, this target is often difficult to achieve. A feasible approach is to allow clear fluids until the child is called into the operating suite. This liberal approach did not lead to an increased incidence of aspiration episodes at a large institution (Andersson *et al.* 2015). Many practitioners, including the author, induce anaesthesia for elective surgery in a child who has drunk a glass of water some minutes before. However, this practice is not yet reflected in the current guidelines.

Finally, the case presented here emphasizes the importance of the presence of an experienced anaesthetist. If a more skilled operator had intubated the trachea correctly on the first attempt, no critical incident would have occurred. In the majority of cases, pulmonary aspiration is not inevitable, but caused by actions of the anaesthetist.

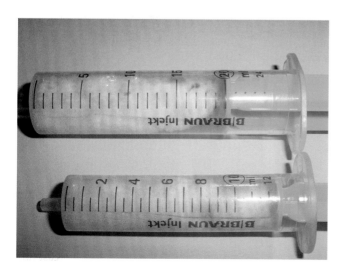

Figure 2.4 A large amount of milk can often be aspirated from the stomach, even when the child is fasted according to protocol.

Summary and Recommendations

This case of complications occurring after an inadequately short fasting time illustrates the importance of a well-functioning organizational process. When anaesthesia is induced earlier than originally planned, the fasting time has to be adapted.

Aspiration of milk is not necessarily a benign event, since it can cause severe disturbance of gas exchange.

In many circumstances, pulmonary aspiration does not occur by chance, but is caused by suboptimal performance on the part of the practitioner.

References

American Society of Anesthesiology (2017). Practice guidelines for preoperative fasting and the use of pharmacologic agents to reduce the risk of pulmonary aspiration: application to healthy patients undergoing elective procedures: an updated report by the American Society of Anesthesiologists Task Force on Preoperative Fasting and the Use of Pharmacologic Agents to Reduce the Risk of Pulmonary Aspiration. *Anesthesiology*, 126, 376–393.

Andersson, H., Zaren, B., & Frykholm, P. (2015). Low incidence of pulmonary aspiration in children allowed intake of clear fluids until called to the operating suite. *Paediatr Anaesth*, 25, 770–777.

Becke, K., Giest, J., & Strauss, J. (2007). Handlungsempfehlungen zur präoperativen Diagnostik, Impfabstand und Nüchternheit im Kindesalter. *Anästh Intensivmed*, 48, S62–S66.

Billeaud, C., Guillet, J., & Sandler, B. (1990). Gastric emptying in infants with or without gastro-oesophageal reflux according to the type of milk. *Eur J Clin Nutr*, 44, 577–583.

Dennhardt, N., Beck, C., Huber, D., *et al.* (2016). Optimized preoperative fasting times decrease ketone body concentration and stabilize mean arterial blood pressure during induction of anesthesia in children younger than 36 months: a prospective observational cohort study. *Paediatr Anaesth*, 26, 838–843.

Engelhardt, T., Wilson, G., Horne, L., *et al.* (2011). Are you hungry? Are you thirsty? Fasting times in elective outpatient pediatric patients. *Paediatr Anaesth*, 21, 964–968.

O'Hare, B., Lerman, J., Endo, J., *et al.* (1996). Acute lung injury after instillation of human breast milk or infant formula into rabbits' lungs. *Anesthesiology*, 84, 1386–1391.

Smith, I., Kranke, P., Murat, I., *et al.* (2011). Perioperative fasting in adults and children: guidelines from the European Society of Anaesthesiology. *Eur J Anaesthesiol*, 28, 556–569.

Soreide, E., Eriksson, L.I., Hirlekar, G., *et al.* (2005). Pre-operative fasting guidelines: an update. *Acta Anaesthesiol Scand*, 49, 1041–1047.

Anticipating Massive Bleeding

Case

Some years ago, a 4 7/12-year-old girl, weighing 20 kg, arrived by air transport. She had fallen while playing in a hayloft and had sustained a penetrating injury from a hayfork in the right supraclavicular region. The mother, a nurse, reported that there had been massive pulsating bleeding and that she had directly called for the helicopter rescue team.

On arrival in the emergency room, the patient was conscious with no active bleeding and only a small 5 mm skin laceration. Wound inspection under general anaesthesia was planned and the patient was brought directly to the operating theatre, where she arrived pale with a blood pressure of 102/64 mmHg and a heart rate of 146 beats per minute. Following intravenous induction, she was intubated and blood was sent by tube mail for crossmatch (retrospectively it became clear that it never arrived in the laboratory). The patient was positioned as for neurosurgery with the anaesthetist at the foot end, with the blood pressure cuff on the right arm and peripheral venous access on the left abducted arm. She was almost completely covered by sterile drapes.

The wound was enlarged by a surgical incision and bleeding reoccurred. Getting a good overview was challenging for the surgical team, which soon included a specialist vascular surgeon, and multiple clamps were placed. The final findings were perforation of the right subclavian artery and the pleura and several lacerated venous vessels.

The child soon became hypotensive, and blood pressure measurements were intermittently unobtainable (retrospectively, because the subclavian artery had been clamped). Attempts for additional venous or arterial access failed, but blood for point-of-care testing could be taken, revealing a haemoglobin concentration of 51 g/l. Finally, although inconvenienced by the surgical drapes, ultrasound-guided femoral artery catheterization was successful and a peripheral venous line on the foot could be placed. At a haemoglobin concentration of 37 g/l, O negative packed red blood cells and fibrinogen was given. After stabilization, the patient was transferred to the paediatric intensive care unit (PICU) still intubated for further care. Ultimately, except for a persistent Horner syndrome, she recovered fully.

Discussion

Hypovolaemia is still one of the leading causes of paediatric cardiac arrest (Bhananker *et al.* 2007). The case presented here is an example of **poor anticipation** and **underestimation of bleeding**, almost ending in disaster. It emphasizes several educational points.

First, **anticipation** of potential surgical complications belongs to the core competencies of the anaesthetist. Stab wounds, especially in the supraclavicular region, are always

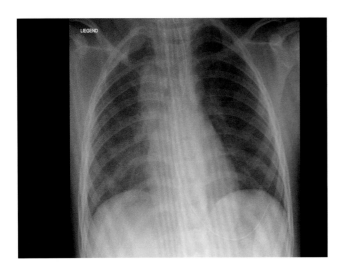

Figure 2.5 Postoperative chest x-ray of the patient, showing a haematoma in the upper mediastinum also displacing the oesophagus to the left.

suspicious, even in the absence of currently active bleeding. Although it seems defensible to start the case with an endotracheal tube (ETT) and a peripheral venous line alone, one should be prepared to gain additional vascular access. Reliable vascular access in both groins would have avoided all access problems. Reduced accessibility in a small patient is a particularity of paediatric anaesthesia. In contrast to adult patients, in whom arterial or central venous access can almost always be inserted during surgery, this is definitely not true for neonates or infants. One has to be prepared beforehand – '**Noah's ark was built before it started to rain**' – and all the drips have to ready.

Second, with a thorough **understanding** of the planned surgical procedure, it would have been foreseeable that surgery might interrupt blood flow to the right arm. The inability to measure the blood pressure should have triggered a view onto the surgical field: undoubtedly, a clamped subclavian artery would then have been suspected. It is probably unfair to blame the surgeon for not spontaneously mentioning this possibility, since the situation was extremely stressful for him as well. Occasionally, the surgeon interrupts important arteries, e.g. the thoracic aorta may be looped before duct ligation and the aortic blood pressure tracing may intermittently disappear; in such situations, oscillometric blood pressure measurement on the right arm can be very helpful and reassuring (cf. Case 2.3). In general, anaesthetists should continuously check the surgical field, as a car driver constantly monitors events on the street.

Third, this case also shows the importance of regular **reassessments**. The plan was to send a blood sample for crossmatch by tube mail to the laboratory. The transport container was placed in the tube mail station, a button was pushed and the person left. More than 90 minutes later, the container was still found undelivered. Therefore, transfusion of non-crossmatched blood was unavoidable. Although the risk of transfusing packed red cells without crossmatch is minimal, exposing the patient to this risk could have been avoided.

In addition, this case illustrates the complexity of **recognizing hypovolaemia** in a child. A normal blood pressure in an awake schoolchild does not exclude severe hypovolaemia. But tachycardia, the patient's pale appearance and the presence of a potentially life-threatening injury should have alarmed the anaesthetist.

In this patient, relevant blood loss could be replaced by crystalloids, packed red blood cells and coagulation factors alone. Fresh frozen plasma is not necessarily needed, and is not very effective for the treatment of dilutional coagulopathy. The first coagulation factor to become critically low is fibrinogen, which can be substituted much more effectively by the administration of fibrinogen (Kozek-Langenecker *et al.* 2017). Over the last decade, the author has completely abandoned the use of fresh frozen plasma outside the field of neonatology, where treatment often takes place in collaboration with a team of neonatologists. Point-of-care coagulation testing, Rotem, has also been used for more than 10 years, but to be honest, in most cases, treatment was initiated first and the Rotem was only used as confirmation of an effective treatment.

Summary and Recommendations

The presented case shows that anticipation of potential bleeding is essential, and that all necessary precautions have to be taken. In small patients, the necessary lines have to be inserted in advance; in older children, access to the potential puncture sites has to be granted.

Surgery can interact with blood pressure or pulse oximetry monitoring when arteries are clamped (cf. Case 2.3). Understanding of the surgical process is needed: always check the surgical field if something unexplained happens.

For the treatment of dilutional coagulopathy, fresh frozen plasma is not essential; in most cases, fibrinogen and later coagulation factors are effective and advantageous.

References

Bhananker, S.M., Ramamoorthy, C., Geiduschek, J.M., *et al.* (2007). Anesthesia-related cardiac arrest in children: update from the Pediatric Perioperative Cardiac Arrest Registry. *Anesth Analg*, 105, 344–350.

Kozek-Langenecker, S.A., Ahmed, A.B., Afshari, A., *et al.* (2017). Management of severe perioperative bleeding: guidelines from the European Society of Anaesthesiology. First update 2016. *Eur J Anaesthesiol*, 34, 332–395.

Maintaining Body Temperature

Case

Many years ago, an 8-year-old girl with cerebral palsy, weighing 14 kg, was scheduled for acetabuloplasty and femoral varus derotation osteotomy because of bilateral hip dislocation. After inhalational induction with sevoflurane and nasotracheal intubation, anaesthesia was maintained with desflurane in air and oxygen. Muscle paralysis was provided by a mivacurium drip. For postoperative analgesia, a caudal block including 40 µg/kg of morphine was performed.

Despite placing her on a forced-air warming mattress right from the beginning, the bladder temperature remained at 34.5 °C for the duration of the procedure (Fig. 2.6). During the intervention, the girl was moved from a left to a right lateral position and then to a supine position for the application of a pelvic cast. After that, she was positioned on the forced-warm-air mattress and a second full-body mattress was placed on top of her using a second warming device. Within 30 minutes core temperature rose to 36.5 °C and desflurane was turned off. The patient was extubated and then transferred to the paediatric intensive care unit (PICU) for further observation.

Discussion

The presented case of a patient with **intraoperative hypothermia** nicely illustrates that it is all about prevention. Hypothermia is typical for children with cerebral palsy (Wongprasartsuk & Stevens 2002) and neurodegenerative diseases (Miao *et al.* 2009) undergoing surgery, because of their reduced metabolic rate ('vita reducta') combined with the large exposure of the body during major orthopaedic interventions. In the author's experience, simply positioning the patient on one forced-warm-air mattress is not sufficient, because the lower part of the body, often up to the mammillary region, is widely exposed during surgery. In addition, during the application of a pelvic cast, a procedure which easily takes an hour or more, the delivery of warmth to the patient is almost impossible. Hypothermia can be prevented by placing a second warming device on top of the patient right from the start and by elevating the room temperature (to e.g. 24 °C). The good news is that when two warming devices are used following surgery the body temperature can reliably be increased to the desired level. However, in the case presented here, hypothermia during surgery may have had a negative impact on the coagulation system or on the infection risk.

Forced-**warm-air devices** have become the universally accepted standard. They are highly effective and complications rarely occur provided the necessary precautions are taken (Azzam & Krock 1995) (cf. Case 8.3). When the body temperature approaches 36.5 °C, the device should be set at 'intermediate' (38 °C) to avoid hyperthermia.

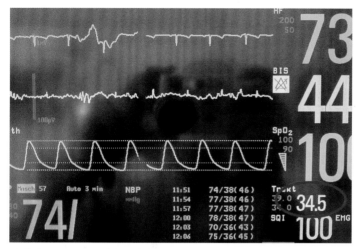

Figure 2.6 This recording is rather typical for a disabled child if no special precautions are taken: hypothermia, bradycardia and low blood pressure.

With adequate **prevention**, profound hypothermia can be avoided. Profound hypothermia can lead to catastrophes. The author remembers the case of a syndromic 5 kg child who was brought to the operating theatre to have a tracheal cannula changed. The procedure was prolonged because of bleeding, bronchoscopy and repeated suctioning. Cardiovascular instability developed resulting in bradycardia. An adrenaline infusion only moderately increased the heart rate. Only at this point was a low body temperature of 32 °C noted. Because of an anticipated short procedure, institutional standards were not followed and the baby was not placed on a forced-warm-air mattress, but only covered with warm towels. Ultimately, with increasing body temperature, the heart rate also increased. Warm towels provide comfort in the awake child, and they can reduce convective losses; however, because of their low specific warmth, cotton towels contribute only marginally to the transfer of heat to the patient. The child has to be covered, but during induction, observation of the thorax is of paramount importance and can be done without negative consequences (Shukry et al. 2012). An additional way to maintain body temperature is the administration of warmed fluids; however, the effectiveness of this should not be overestimated, because with the low flow rates used in paediatric patients the warmed fluids will have reached room temperature by the time they enter the body (Bissonnette & Paut 2002).

The prevention of hypothermia necessitates **measuring temperature**. In the author's practice, a lower oesophageal temperature probe combined with the oesophageal stethoscope was used in intubated children. Measuring the temperature via a gastric tube or an indwelling bladder catheter is very convenient; however, with an open abdomen, the values may not correctly reflect core body temperature. In all other cases, tympanal (intermittently) or rectal probes (continuously) were used. In any case, temperature has to be measured and recorded in every anaesthetized child.

A special situation is **MRI examination**. Hypothermia is typically not a problem, because the MRI causes an increase in temperature in the examined tissues (Bryan et al. 2006, Lo et al. 2014). This warming effect is more pronounced in a 3 tesla MRI device (Machata et al. 2009). Radiologists fear hyperthermia; but, in reality, because of the cold environment in the scanning room, body temperature is usually just maintained and active warming is usually not required.

During anaesthesia, the body regulates its temperature in a much wider range. When a large part of the body is covered and only a small part is exposed during prolonged surgery, e.g. in **ENT surgery**, body temperature starts to rise after some time and hyperthermia is regularly encountered. This is due to the highly active metabolism and the large endogenous heat production in children. Consequently, active warming is usually not indicated in such cases.

Summary and Recommendations

With adequate prevention, profound hypothermia can usually be avoided. Today, the use of forced-warm-air devices has become the standard.

Children with cerebral palsy or neurodegenerative disorders rapidly develop hypothermia because of their reduced metabolism.

References

Azzam, F.J. & Krock, J.L. (1995). Thermal burns in two infants associated with a forced air warming system. *Anesth Analg*, 81, 661.

Bissonnette, B. & Paut, O. (2002). Active warming of saline or blood is ineffective when standard infusion tubing is used: an experimental study. *Can J Anaesth*, 49, 270–275.

Bryan, Y.F., Templeton, T.W., Nick, T.G., *et al.* (2006). Brain magnetic resonance imaging increases core body temperature in sedated children. *Anesth Analg*, 102, 1674–1679.

Lo, C., Ormond, G., McDougall, R., Sheppard, S.J., *et al.* (2014). Effect of magnetic resonance imaging on core body temperature in anaesthetised children. *Anaesth Intensive Care*, 42, 333–339.

Machata, A.M., Willschke, H., Kabon, B., *et al.* (2009). Effect of brain magnetic resonance imaging on body core temperature in sedated infants and children. *Br J Anaesth*, 102, 385–389.

Miao, N., Levin, S.W., Baker, E.H., *et al.* (2009). Children with infantile neuronal ceroid lipofuscinosis have an increased risk of hypothermia and bradycardia during anesthesia. *Anesth Analg*, 109, 372–378.

Shukry, M., Matthews, L., de Armendi, A.J., *et al.* (2012). Does the covering of children during induction of anesthesia have an effect on body temperature at the end of surgery? *J Clin Anesth*, 24, 116–120.

Wongprasartsuk, P. & Stevens, J. (2002). Cerebral palsy and anaesthesia. *Paediatr Anaesth*, 12, 296–303.

Case 2.7

Unexpected Laboratory Results

Case

A 15-month-old boy, weighing 9 kg, was scheduled for epispadias repair, an extensive urological intervention with only minimal blood loss and an approximate duration of 4 hours. After inhalational induction and securing the airway, the cephalic vein at left forearm was cannulated with a 24G cannula under ultrasound guidance. This cannula was replaced via a guidewire by a 2F catheter with a length of 5 cm. Ringer's lactate containing 1% glucose was started at a maintenance rate. In addition, a 24G 18 mm cannula was inserted into the left external jugular vein for repeated blood sampling (Fig. 2.7). A blood sample taken immediately after insertion showed moderate hypercarbia but otherwise normal values (Table 2.7).

Surgery started with the uneventful insertion of a large suprapubic catheter, with moderate bleeding. Two boluses of a crystalloid solution were given and dopamine was started at an initial rate of 10 µg/kg/min to maintain a mean arterial blood pressure of at least 45 mmHg. Two hours after skin incision, a routine blood sample was drawn from the external jugular catheter with the following results: haemoglobin 55 g/l, pH 7.22, lactate 13.4 mmol/l, glucose 25.0 mmol/l (Table 2.7). The anaesthetist was very surprised and tried to find possible explanations for these unexpected findings. A repeat sample showed almost identical results.

A wide differential diagnosis was considered. The surgeon examined the abdomen to rule out bleeding or intestinal laceration caused by the insertion of the large suprapubic catheter. Finally, an arterial catheter was inserted for blood pressure monitoring and repeated blood sampling. An arterial blood sample now showed normal values.

Discussion

This case illustrates the possibility of **spurious laboratory results**, which are not obvious at a first glance. This unexpected result, showing anaemia and massively elevated lactate and glucose levels, unsettled the whole team. A second blood sample, which was taken after withdrawing (and later reinjecting) 10 ml of the patient's blood, showed identical results. The hypothesis of infusion solution admixture was rejected at first because the sampling catheter was at the neck and the infusion line in the forearm. In addition, the initial blood sample taken from the same line had shown normal results.

The **differential diagnosis** should always consider medical conditions first. A number of possibilities, including the following, were evaluated. An intra-abdominal laceration caused by the insertion of the suprapubic drainage, leading to blood loss, intestinal ischaemia and elevated lactate, was not supported by the patient's stable haemodynamic course and

Table 2.7 Laboratory results obtained during epispadias repair

	Venous blood sample after induction (spontaneous ventilation)	Venous blood sample at 2 hours of surgery	Arterial blood sample at 3 hours of surgery
pH	7.22	7.22	7.31
pCO_2	8.23 kPa	4.43 kPa	6.12 kPa
Haemoglobin	118 g/l	**55 g/l**	95 g/l
Base excess	−2.4	**−12.8**	−2.7
Lactate	1.5 mmol/l	**13.4 mmol/l**	2.5 mmol/l
Glucose	6.3 mmol/l	**25.0 mmol/l**	7.3 mmol/l

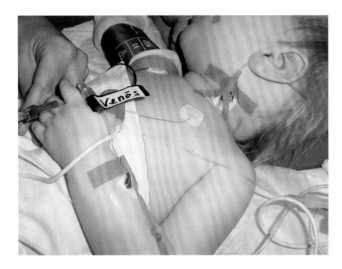

Figure 2.7 This 24G 18 mm venous catheter in the external jugular vein was used for blood sampling; there was no running infusion.

normal abdominal palpation. Malignant hyperthermia seemed very unlikely, because elevated lactate levels are a very late event and there were no signs of hypermetabolism; in addition, this would not explain the anaemia (Rosenberg *et al.* 2015). The combination of hyperglycaemia and elevated lactate is not typical for perioperative decompensation of the common inherited metabolic diseases, e.g. acyl CoA dehydrogenase deficiencies (Allen *et al.* 2017).

Wrong measurements due to inadequate **sampling technique** commonly include elevated potassium concentrations in a haemolytic sample or metabolic acidosis secondary to the admixture of too much heparin to a blood gas syringe (Ordog *et al.* 1985). In this case, an arterial line was inserted and the blood sample now showed normal values (Table 2.7). The final interpretation in the presented case was **admixture** of infusion solution to the blood sample. The external jugular vein usually runs into the subclavian vein; however, many variations exist. Surprisingly, in this tiny patient, even an 18 mm cannula inserted at the neck must have reached the subclavian vein when the shoulder was elevated. Therefore, the blood sample reflected a 1:1 mixture of patient's blood and Ringer's lactate.

Spurious readings caused by admixture also can occur with **capnography**. When there is a leak in the sampling line, measured end-tidal gas concentrations are falsely low. If this error is not recognized, the anaesthetist will reduce the minute ventilation and cause hypoventilation. Falsely low readings of the anaesthetic gas will trigger an anaesthetic overdose.

Summary and Recommendations

The presented case of spurious laboratory results of a sample taken from an external jugular vein shows that infusion solution admixture may not be obvious at a first glance.

It is important to always exclude potentially severe medical conditions first, before classifying unexpected results as 'fake news'.

Falsification of laboratory results by admixture and dilution of a blood or gas sample is a common error in clinical practice.

In general, for major surgery, it may be prudent to have an arterial or central venous line for reliable repeated blood sampling.

References

Allen, C., Perkins, R., & Schwahn, B. (2017). A retrospective review of anesthesia and perioperative care in children with medium-chain acyl-CoA dehydrogenase deficiency. *Paediatr Anaesth*, 27, 60–65.

Ordog, G.J., Wasserberger, J., & Balasubramaniam, S. (1985). Effect of heparin on arterial blood gases. *Ann Emerg Med*, 14, 233–238.

Rosenberg, H., Pollock, N., Schiemann, A., *et al.* (2015). Malignant hyperthermia: a review. *Orphanet J Rare Dis*, 10, 93.

3 Airway-Related Problems

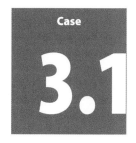

Breathing System

Case 3.1

Case

A long time ago, a 3-year-old girl, weighing 14 kg, was scheduled for inguinal hernia repair. Despite rectal premedication with midazolam 14 mg, she was still very active and refused to lie down on the operating table. Parental presence was not yet standard at that time. The decision of the team was to induce anaesthesia in a sitting position by mask using a Bain circuit. Nitrous oxide 60% was administered, followed by sevoflurane 8%.

The charismatic anaesthetist talked to her, suggesting that she could now fall into a good sleep with nice dreams, and indeed she followed his suggestion, closed her eyes and her muscle tone got weaker. About 1 minute later, her respiratory rate increased, she started to move, suddenly opened her eyes and shoved the mask away.

It was now realized that she had never received an anaesthetic gas because the switch on the anaesthesia machine was turned towards 'circle system' and not to 'open system'. Hypnosis was induced only by the suggestive words of the anaesthetist until continuous rebreathing created hypercarbia, made her uncomfortable and finally woke her up.

Discussion

This case of **failed anaesthesia induction** because of a faulty action by the anaesthetist illustrates the importance of meticulously checking the anaesthesia machine before every case. The author has seen this mistake – selecting the **wrong anaesthetic system** – in many dozens of cases during his career (Fig. 3.1). When an inhalational induction is planned and no gas arrives at the mask end of the circuit, the consequence will be mild: the child simply does not go to sleep. The situation is much worse when an intravenous induction is performed. The child will then be connected to the wrong circuit and fruitless efforts to ventilate the lungs with the other system will follow. The author is aware of such a case, which led to profound hypoxaemia, the misdiagnosis of bronchospasm and tube exchange before the mistake was recognized. Fortunately, no long-term sequelae occurred. It should be highlighted that failure to measure exhaled CO_2 and sevoflurane concentrations, which was seen in the presented case, should always be considered a warning sign. Admittedly, during induction the most common cause for this phenomenon is insufficient tightness of the face mask, especially when a double mask scavenging system is used, but other possibilities should always be considered as well.

There is still debate about the **optimal anaesthesia system for induction**. A **circle system** is almost uniformly used for maintenance of anaesthesia in children. Fresh gas use can be minimized to far less than one litre per minute and waste gas scavenging is improved. In addition, modern coaxial tubing systems, even with an integrated

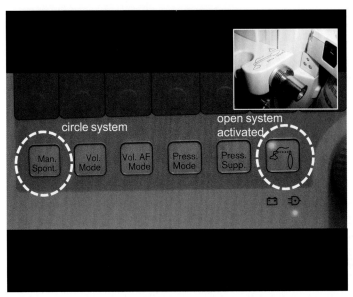

circle system

open system activated

Man. Spont.

Vol. Mode

Vol. AF Mode

Press. Mode

Press. Supp.

Figure 3.1 An anaesthesia machine allowing the use of a circle system as well as an open system, e.g. a Jackson Rees modification of a T-piece.

capnography sampling tube, have made the system handier and much less bulky. On the other hand, the lightweight open anaesthesia system, e.g. the **Jackson Rees modification of the T-piece** (Jackson Rees 1950), with no valves, which allows rapid changes in the inspiratory gas composition, is an attractive option for anaesthesia induction in children. Until recently, such systems were widely used by British (Marsh & Mackie 2009) as well as French (Fesseau *et al.* 2014) paediatric anaesthetists. The compact size and ease of use are probably the major reasons for this preference (Meakin 2007). On the other hand, with the circle system, the novice has a steeper learning curve and unintended high airway pressures with gastric insufflation can more easily be avoided (von Ungern-Sternberg *et al.* 2007). It is debatable if one or the other system allows better recognition of changes in compliance during manual ventilation; it is likely that the experience of the practitioner is the most important factor in this regard (Schily *et al.* 2001).

The author is convinced that the trend towards the uniform use of circle systems for induction as well as for maintenance of anaesthesia will continue, mainly because the advantages of using an open system are not really evident, and because modern circle systems allow the continuous measurement of flows and pressures. In addition, the presence of a pressure release valve set at 13 cmH$_2$O allows avoiding gastric insufflation, and waste gas scavenging diminishes pollution of the theatre. However, even with modern anaesthesia machines, a second outlet in addition to the circle system is desirable in order to be able to administer tailored gas mixtures and not only 100% oxygen, e.g. by nasal cannula or by face mask.

Faulty manipulations by the anaesthetist are a major cause of complications. In order to make the equipment more resilient against wrong manipulations, many institutions, including the author's, have eliminated the possibility of switching between two anaesthetic circuits. However, many sources for mistakes still remain; a typical one is **incorrect**

connection of the tubing after accidental disconnection. When the expiratory limb is connected to the outlet designated for the bag, massive inflation of the patient's lungs can occur, with the risk of barotrauma and cardiocirculatory collapse. The author has witnessed several such events during his professional career and wonders why the industry has not yet eliminated this possibility by using different connectors for the inspiratory and expiratory limbs, and especially for the tubing for the bag.

Historically, it was recommended – also to the author when he was a novice – to always smell at the mask before placing it over the face of the child. In the case presented here, the absence of any gas flow would have been noted, and would have prevented this complication. Sniffing anaesthetic gases does not fit well with today's fear of operating room pollution and the conviction that even traces of anaesthetic gases are harmful (Meier *et al.* 1995). Nevertheless, ensuring that fresh gas really reaches the child is still a prerequisite for successful anaesthesia induction.

Summary and Recommendations

This case of failed anaesthesia induction because a switch on the anaesthesia machine was in the wrong position emphasizes the importance of a meticulous equipment check.

Real failure of the anaesthesia machine is an extremely rare event; faulty manipulations by the anaesthetist are much more common.

References

Fesseau, R., Alacoque, X., Larcher, C., et al. (2014). An ADARPEF survey on respiratory management in pediatric anesthesia. *Paediatr Anaesth*, 24, 1099–1105.

Jackson Rees, G. (1950). Anaesthesia in the newborn. *Br Med J*, 2 (4694), 1419–1422.

Marsh, D.F. & Mackie, P. (2009). National survey of pediatric breathing systems use in the UK. *Paediatr Anaesth*, 19, 477–480.

Meakin, G.H. (2007). Role of the Jackson Rees T-piece in pediatric anesthesia. *Paediatr Anaesth*, 17, 613–615.

Meier, A., Jost, M., Ruegger, et al. (1995). Narcotic gas burden of personnel in pediatric anesthesia [in German]. *Anaesthesist*, 44, 154–162.

Schily, M., Koumoukelis, H., Lerman, J., et al. (2001). Can pediatric anesthesiologists detect an occluded tracheal tube in neonates? *Anesth Analg*, 93, 66–70.

von Ungern-Sternberg, B.S., Saudan, S., Regli, A., et al. (2007). Should the use of modified Jackson Rees T-piece breathing system be abandoned in preschool children? *Paediatr Anaesth*, 17, 654–660.

Case

A 9-month-old girl with a Pierre Robin sequence, weighing 8 kg, was scheduled for cleft palate repair. The child was induced by mask with sevoflurane and nitrous oxide. After neuromuscular blockade, the trachea was intubated uneventfully via a laryngeal mask airway (LMA) size 1.5 with the aid of a 2.2 mm bronchoscope and a mounted size 3.5 uncuffed endotracheal tube (ETT). The uncuffed tube was then replaced with a 3.5 RAE Microcuff ETT via a 7F Cook airway exchanger.

Anaesthesia was maintained with sevoflurane, repeated doses of fentanyl, and dexmede-tomidine 0.5 µg/kg/h as a co-analgesic agent. At the end of surgery, the child was extubated and noted to have noisy breathing but otherwise no visible signs of airway obstruction. The child was transferred to the intensive care unit, and 20 hours later to the regular ward.

During the second postoperative night, 36 hours after surgery, signs of upper airway obstruction with stridor and the need for supplementary oxygen developed. The child was transferred to the intensive care unit. Despite 100% oxygen by face mask and a jaw thrust manoeuvre to open the airway, oxygen saturation dropped below 80% and an emergency call was sent out. The anaesthetist on call successfully managed the situation by inserting an LMA Supreme size 1.5. Copious secretions were noted. Morphine and midazolam were given to the struggling child, and the team waited for the arrival of the senior paediatric anaesthetist.

He tried a fibreoptic intubation through the correctly positioned LMA Supreme; there was a good view, but as could be expected, intubation was not possible through this type of LMA. Direct laryngoscopy was unsuccessful. The LMA Supreme was replaced with a classic type. The fibreoptic bronchoscope easily passed the cords, but while railroading the ETT severe laryngospasm occurred. Rocuronium 1 mg/kg was given, but ventilation remained unsuccessful. The child now became bradycardic, and chest compressions were started. Atropine and two doses of 10 µg/kg adrenaline were given. Foamy secretions emerging from the LMA impeded the next attempt at fibreoptic intubation. At this point, the senior nurse proposed proceeding to a surgical airway. The senior staff anaesthetist, however, decided to make one further attempt at fibreoptic intubation through the LMA. After repeatedly suctioning the airway, this was finally successful.

The child remained intubated for 9 days, but left the hospital without any long-term sequelae.

Discussion

This is a 'cannot intubate, cannot ventilate' situation in a child with a Pierre Robin sequence and, therefore, expected to be difficult to intubate. In the elective situation on the day of surgery, intubation was completely uneventful, primarily using the fibreoptic approach via an LMA (Jöhr & Berger 2004). In the emergency situation in the intensive care unit, upper airway obstruction combined with copious secretions and impaired gas exchange almost led to a fatal outcome. It remained unclear what caused delayed airway obstruction after cleft palate repair, but inflammatory swelling was the most likely explanation.

Insertion of an LMA should be an early step in a 'cannot intubate, cannot ventilate' situation (Weiss & Engelhardt 2010). In the presented case, it did not provide a perfect airway, but was sufficient to keep the girl alive. Fibreoptic intubation via an LMA is a standard procedure in children, and every anaesthetist should be familiar with it. Blind intubation through an LMA is nearly always unsuccessful and should not be attempted (Kleine-Brueggeney *et al.* 2015).

The presented case also illustrates the importance of preventing functional airway obstruction, such as laryngospasm. If a muscle relaxant had been given prior to the first intubation attempt, the near-fatal situation could have been avoided (Weiss & Engelhardt 2012). When everything else fails, a surgical airway should be considered, as suggested by the nurse in this case. Unfortunately, even in animal (Holm-Knudsen *et al.* 2012) or in human adult cadavers (Heymans *et al.* 2016) a cannula technique has a high failure rate and cannot be recommended for emergency situations (Duggan *et al.* 2016). In a neonate or a small infant, a front neck access is a very demanding procedure; the cricothyroid membrane, on the other hand, will be large enough to allow the passage of an ETT, as demonstrated by a serious adverse event described in Case 3.7.

Every practitioner should know the algorithm to manage a 'cannot intubate, cannot ventilate' situation by heart. A guideline is like the score for the conductor of an orchestra: you can choose to make variations. In the presented clinical situation, the anaesthetist decided to continue with fibreoptic intubation and not, as proposed by the guideline, to perform a front neck access, because he was convinced he would be able to perform intubation by this technique.

The **Pierre Robin sequence** is characterized by micrognathia, glossoptosis (Fig. 3.2) and airway obstruction. A cleft palate is common, but does not occur in all patients with a Pierre Robin sequence (Cladis *et al.* 2014). Typically, neonates present with signs and symptoms of upper airway obstruction and feeding difficulties. In mild cases, airway obstruction can be overcome by positioning the infant in a prone position; in more severe cases, surgical interventions are needed, e.g. glossopexy (Fujii *et al.* 2015), tracheotomy or mandibular distraction. Airway management is often challenging. It can usually be secured easily with an LMA, whereas laryngoscopy is difficult. A paraglossal approach enhances the view in most patients, and video laryngoscopy has greatly facilitated intubation of these patients. Of course, fibreoptic intubation via an LMA in the anaesthetized child is a very valuable option.

Summary and Recommendations

This case of a 'cannot intubate, cannot ventilate' situation emphasizes the importance of being familiar with relevant algorithms.

Fibreoptic intubation via an LMA is a standard technique in paediatric anaesthesia which should be taught and practised.

Every guideline has room for some variation. It is like a recipe, which is usually followed, but from which the cook can deviate if the situation justifies it.

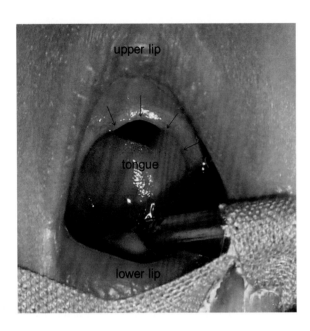

Figure 3.2 A neonate with a Pierre Robin sequence; the tongue has fallen backwards and downwards; it is now behind the cleft (arrows) and obstructs the airway.

References

Cladis, F., Kumar, A., Grunwaldt, L., *et al.* (2014). Pierre Robin sequence: a perioperative review. *Anesth Analg*, 119, 400–412.

Duggan, L.V., Ballantyne, S.B., Law, J.A., *et al.* (2016). Transtracheal jet ventilation in the 'can't intubate can't oxygenate' emergency: a systematic review. *Br J Anaesth*, 117 (Suppl. 1), i28–i38.

Fujii, M., Tachibana, K., Takeuchi, M., *et al.* (2015). Perioperative management of 19 infants undergoing glossopexy (tongue–lip adhesion) procedure: a retrospective study. *Paediatr Anaesth*, 25, 829–833.

Heymans, F., Feigl, G., Graber, S., *et al.* (2016). Emergency cricothyrotomy performed by surgical airway-naive medical personnel: a randomized crossover study in cadavers comparing three commonly used techniques. *Anesthesiology*, 125, 295–303.

Holm-Knudsen, R.J., Rasmussen, L.S., Charabi, B., *et al.* (2012). Emergency airway access in children: transtracheal cannulas and tracheotomy assessed in a porcine model. *Paediatr Anaesth*, 22, 1159–1165.

Jöhr, M. & Berger, T.M. (2004). Fiberoptic intubation through the laryngeal mask airway (LMA) as a standardized procedure. *Paediatr Anaesth*, 14, 614.

Kleine-Brueggeney, M., Nicolet, A., Nabecker, S., *et al.* (2015). Blind intubation of anaesthetised children with supraglottic airway devices AmbuAura-i and Air-Q cannot be recommended: a randomised controlled trial. *Eur J Anaesthesiol*, 32, 631–639.

Weiss, M. & Engelhardt, T. (2010). Proposal for the management of the unexpected difficult pediatric airway. *Paediatr Anaesth*, 20, 454–464.

Weiss, M. & Engelhardt, T. (2012). Cannot ventilate: paralyze! *Paediatr Anaesth*, 22, 1147–1149.

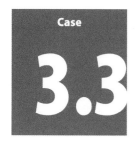

Can Intubate, Cannot Ventilate

Case

A 5-month-old girl, weighing 4.8 kg, was scheduled for oesophageal dilatation under general anaesthesia. Previously, a long gap oesophageal atresia had been repaired elsewhere. There was a functioning gastrostomy. Endotracheal intubation was reported to be difficult.

After premedication with atropine 30 µg/kg via gastrostomy to reduce the abundant oral secretions, anaesthesia was induced by mask. The child was paralysed with mivacurium 0.2 mg/kg, ventilated with the anaesthesia machine, and successfully intubated with a cuffed size 3.0 endotracheal tube (ETT) using fibreoptic guidance and the Frei endoscopy mask. Oesophageal dilatation was begun with a size 14F dilator and increased stepwise. After insertion of a size 22F dilator, ventilation suddenly became impossible even with a peak pressure of 20 cmH$_2$O. When the dilator was removed, expiratory CO$_2$ immediately reappeared (Fig. 3.3).

Obviously, despite correct position of the ETT, the presence of a large foreign body in the oesophagus led to a complete obstruction of the tracheal lumen.

Discussion

This case illustrates a typical '**can intubate, cannot ventilate**' situation, where the ETT is in place but ventilation is still not possible. In this case, the experienced team immediately realized that the large dilator in the oesophagus caused the complete obstruction of the trachea, which was immediately reversed when the instrument was taken out. Airway obstruction is a typical complication of oesophageal dilatation (Gercek *et al.* 2007) or of transoesophageal echocardiography in infants when large devices are used (Andropoulos *et al.* 2000). In preterm babies weighing less than 800 g, even a 9F oesophageal stethoscope can completely impede ventilation. The author has also seen severe airway obstruction in a toddler when a piece of apple got stuck in the oesophagus.

The '**cannot intubate, cannot ventilate**' situation (cf. Case 3.2) is obviously also a dramatic event, but the practitioner can follow an accepted algorithm down to the final step of a surgical airway, when everything else fails (Weiss & Engelhardt 2010). In contrast, if ventilation is impossible after successful intubation (i.e. the '**can intubate, cannot ventilate**' situation), finding a solution can be much more demanding. Functional problems, such as superficial anaesthesia or insufficient neuromuscular blockade, are common and have to be excluded (Weiss & Engelhardt 2012). The initial steps are clear: the function of the anaesthesia ventilator and a free passage of a suction catheter through the ETT can be rapidly assessed, but then several scenarios are possible and successful treatment requires a correct diagnosis. Knowledge of the patient's past medical history, physical findings, and

(a)

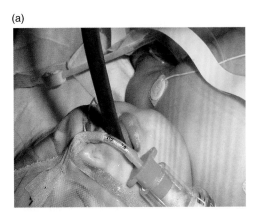

Figure 3.3 (a) A large oesophageal bougie completely obstructs the airway in a small infant, and (b) expiratory CO_2 disappears.

(b)

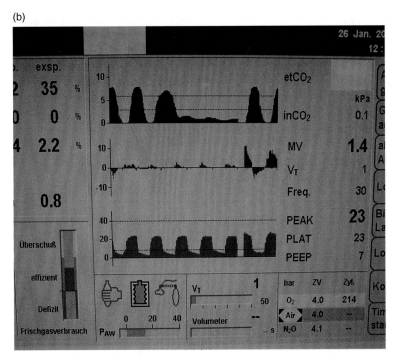

often some intuition as well, may be crucial. The differential diagnosis includes but is not limited to compression of the airway, main-stem intubation, position of the tip of the ETT in a fistula, severe bronchospasm, as well as external compression of the lung by tension pneumothorax, gastric distension (Berg *et al.* 1998) or a large mediastinal mass (Pearson & Tan 2015).

Typically, rather dramatic situations occur during a **percutaneous gastrostomy** procedure in small children. The gastrostomy tube is pulled down the oesophagus until it exits through the abdominal wall. Usually, a strong resistance is felt when the bulky part of the tube passes the middle portion of the oesophagus right behind the carina, and sometimes completely compresses the airway. An inexperienced anaesthetist might advise the surgeon to interrupt the procedure because ventilation has become impossible. But this will in fact put the patient at an even greater risk, because there is only one solution to this problem: the gastrostomy tube has to be pulled down completely; there is no way back.

Summary and Recommendations

The presented case shows that a large foreign body in the oesophagus can compress the airway and completely impede ventilation.

Managing the 'can intubate, cannot ventilate' situation is challenging. While following the steps of an algorithm can be helpful, thereafter, only the correct diagnosis can save the life of the child.

References

Andropoulos, D.B., Ayres, N.A., Stayer, S.A., et al. (2000). The effect of transesophageal echocardiography on ventilation in small infants undergoing cardiac surgery. *Anesth Analg*, 90, 47–49.

Berg, M.D., Idris, A.H., & Berg, R.A. (1998). Severe ventilatory compromise due to gastric distention during pediatric cardiopulmonary resuscitation. *Resuscitation*, 36, 71–73.

Gercek, A., Ay, B., Dogan, V., *et al.* (2007). Esophageal balloon dilation in children: prospective analysis of hemodynamic changes and complications during general anesthesia. *J Clin Anesth*, 19, 286–289.

Pearson, J.K. & Tan, G.M. (2015). Pediatric anterior mediastinal mass: a review article. *Semin Cardiothorac Vasc Anesth*, 19, 248–254.

Weiss, M. & Engelhardt, T. (2010). Proposal for the management of the unexpected difficult pediatric airway. *Paediatr Anaesth*, 20, 454–464.

Weiss, M. & Engelhardt, T. (2012). Cannot ventilate: paralyze! *Paediatr Anaesth*, 22, 1147–1149.

Laryngospasm

Case

A long time ago, a 2-year-old girl (body weight 12 kg) presented with a lip laceration that required surgical repair. She was premedicated with 10 mg (0.8 mg/kg) of rectal midazolam, an intravenous line was inserted and 20 mg (1.7 mg/kg) of racemic ketamine was given. Standard monitoring was applied.

While the surgeon was cleaning the lip and exploring the field, the anaesthetist filled out the anaesthesia protocol. Suddenly, he heard the oxygen saturation decreasing; when he turned to the patient, he noticed deeply cyanotic lips and tried to ventilate her by mask, which proved to be impossible because of a rigid abdomen. Next, the heart rate decreased and for a full width of the scope there was no QRS complex visible. He immediately advised the nurse to start chest compressions. During cardiac massage, 20 mg (1.7 mg/kg) of succinylcholine was injected, followed by atropine 0.25 mg (0.02 mg/kg). Mask ventilation was then successful, the heart rate picked up, the trachea was intubated with a size 5.0 uncuffed endotracheal tube, and surgery was completed.

The girl made an uneventful recovery and left the hospital 2 hours after surgery.

Discussion

This case illustrates how an **inattentive anaesthetist**, overlooking the early warning signs (irregular breathing and slight coughing), can be taken aback by **laryngospasm**. Even though those warning signs are almost always present, this anaesthetist became aware of the situation only when the child was already deeply cyanotic. Earlier intervention with opening up the airway, applying positive airway pressure and inducing muscle relaxation when needed would almost certainly have avoided **cardiac arrest**. Laryngospasm is still a major cause of cardiac arrest, especially in otherwise healthy children (Morray et al. 2000, Ramamoorthy et al. 2010). The prevention seems to be very simple: the presence of an attentive and skilled anaesthetist.

The **pathophysiology** of laryngospasm is still poorly understood. In the presence of light planes of anaesthesia, a normally protective airway reflex can turn into an exaggerated reaction potentially leading to organ damage. Laryngospasm is less likely to occur when airway instrumentation, especially endotracheal intubation, is avoided. It is still a matter of debate whether airway removal is better done when the patient is awake or asleep. Extubation or removal of a laryngeal mask airway (LMA) under deep anaesthesia clearly reduces the occurrence of laryngospasm; it is still possible, however, that severe laryngospasm occurs many minutes later. This highlights the fact that children have to be monitored in the recovery area until they are fully awake. The use of propofol is associated with a lower risk of laryngospasm compared to sevoflurane, and desflurane should probably best be avoided. Lidocaine, intravenously or topically, has been shown to protect against the occurrence of laryngospasm (Mihara *et al.* 2014). It was the author's practice to administer lidocaine 1–2 mg/kg intravenously in patients at high risk, e.g. before the second trial of extubation after a previous episode of laryngospasm leading to re-intubation.

Respiratory complications, such as laryngospasm, are more common in younger patients (Habre *et al.* 2017, von Ungern-Sternberg *et al.* 2010). They occur more frequently with less experienced anaesthetists and when a child is suffering from a current or recent (within 2 weeks of surgery) upper respiratory infection (von Ungern-Sternberg *et al.* 2010). Infants with respiratory syncytium virus (RSV) infection seem to be at an extremely high risk (Wörner *et al.* 2009). It was the practice of the author to premedicate patients with an upper respiratory infection and abundant secretions with atropine 30–40 µg/kg orally or rectally, usually 30–40 minutes before the induction of anaesthesia; admittedly, scientific proof supporting this measure is relatively weak (Shaw *et al.* 2000), but nevertheless it appeared to be very effective.

Ketamine is widely used by anaesthetists and by emergency physicians to provide deep sedation – perhaps better called general anaesthesia because the child is intended to be non-reactive to pain – for skin laceration repair or other minor interventions (Fig. 3.4). Overall, ketamine is considered to be a safe compound, but respiratory complications such as laryngospasm are always a threat (Gloor *et al.* 2001, Melendez & Bachur 2009). Co-administration of atropine reduces secretions, but not the incidence of respiratory complications (Kye *et al.* 2012). Ketamine almost guarantees haemodynamic stability, even in vulnerable patients, and an open airway is spontaneously maintained. Intact airway reflexes protect from aspiration, but enhance the occurrence of coughing and laryngospasm. The presence of an attentive physician is obviously mandatory.

Summary and Recommendations

This case emphasizes that ketamine sedation needs continuous careful surveillance and a high index of suspicion for potential complications.

Airway obstruction and laryngospasm require immediate intervention, and equipment and drugs must be ready for use: mask, bag and oxygen as well as a muscle relaxant drawn up in a syringe.

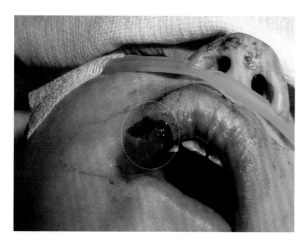

Figure 3.4 Laceration of the lip needing a few surgical stitches. A single dose of ketamine and an open airway seems to be an easy approach; however, severe airway complications, such as laryngospasm, can occur.

References

Gloor, A., Dillier, C., & Gerber, A. (2001). Ketamine for short ambulatory procedures in children: an audit. *Paediatr Anaesth*, 11, 533–539.

Habre, W., Disma, N., Virag, K., *et al.* (2017). Incidence of severe critical events in paediatric anaesthesia (APRICOT): a prospective multicentre observational study in 261 hospitals in Europe. *Lancet Respir Med*, 5, 412–425.

Kye, Y.C., Rhee, J.E., Kim, K., *et al.* (2012). Clinical effects of adjunctive atropine during ketamine sedation in pediatric emergency patients. *Am J Emerg Med*, 30, 1981–1985.

Melendez, E. & Bachur, R. (2009). Serious adverse events during procedural sedation with ketamine. *Pediatr Emerg Care*, 25, 325–328.

Mihara, T., Uchimoto, K., Morita, S., *et al.* (2014). The efficacy of lidocaine to prevent laryngospasm in children: a systematic review and meta-analysis. *Anaesthesia*, 69, 1388–1396.

Morray, J.P., Geiduschek, J.M., Ramamoorthy, C., *et al.* (2000). Anesthesia-related cardiac arrest in children: initial findings of the Pediatric Perioperative Cardiac Arrest (POCA) Registry. *Anesthesiology*, 93, 6–14.

Ramamoorthy, C., Haberkern, C.M., Bhananker, S.M., *et al.* (2010). Anesthesia-related cardiac arrest in children with heart disease: data from the Pediatric Perioperative Cardiac Arrest (POCA) Registry. *Anesth Analg*, 110, 1376–1382.

Shaw, C.A., Kelleher, A.A., Gill, C.P., *et al.* (2000). Comparison of the incidence of complications at induction and emergence in infants receiving oral atropine vs no premedication. *Br J Anaesth*, 84, 174–178.

von Ungern-Sternberg, B.S., Boda, K., Chambers, N.A., *et al.* (2010). Risk assessment for respiratory complications in paediatric anaesthesia: a prospective cohort study. *Lancet*, 376, 773–783.

Wörner, J., Jöhr, M., Berger, T.M., *et al.* (2009). Infections with respiratory syncytial virus. Underestimated risk during anaesthesia in infants [in German]. *Anaesthesist*, 58, 1041–1044.

Inappropriately Sized Endotracheal Tube

Case

A long time ago, a 10-month-old girl was scheduled for a further session of staged resection of a congenital naevus covering large parts of the trunk. She had previously undergone several uneventful anaesthetics. After a halothane induction and neuromuscular paralysis, a size 4.0 uncuffed endotracheal tube (ETT) was inserted. Because of inappropriately high leakage, the decision was made to replace the ETT with a larger one. The size 4.5 ETT only passed with significant resistance. It was nevertheless left in place because the leak with the smaller ETT was thought to make ventilation unreliable given the patient's prone position with limited access to the head. Cuffed ETTs for infants were not yet routinely available. Recovery was uneventful with the exception of a mild post-extubation stridor, which was treated with moist air.

At the time of the next anaesthetic, at the age of 14 months, a size 4.0 uncuffed ETT provided a perfect fit with no leak. Even at the age of 2 years, only a size 4.0 ETT passed without resistance. At this age, fibreoptic inspection showed moderate subglottic narrowing. The child remained asymptomatic. Later, with increasing growth, larger ETTs could be used but always had to be chosen at least two sizes below the age-based calculated size.

Discussion

This is the only case of **subglottic stenosis** following short-term intubation encountered by the author during his 40-year career. It is very likely that the forceful passage of the inappropriately sized ETT caused some damage, inflammation and scarring. It is very likely that the use of a correctly sized cuffed ETT (i.e. a size 3.5 for this 10-month-old girl) would have allowed ventilation of the child and avoided the damage. Fortunately, the consequences were mild in this case, with post-extubation stridor as the only symptom and no limitations of her daily life. At that date, when uncuffed tubes were usually used, it was the author's practice to perform a fibreoptic exam whenever an ETT with a correct fit was two sizes smaller than predicted by age-based formulas, mainly to identify pre-existing pathologies such as a subglottic haemangioma.

There is no doubt that **inappropriately large ETTs** can cause damage to the subglottic region and must be avoided under all circumstances. Traditional teaching was that a moderate leak should be present at airway pressures exceeding 25 cmH$_2$O when uncuffed ETTs were used; with a cuffed ETT, a leak should always be present with the non-inflated cuff. When using a cuffed ETT, the cuff should never be positioned at the level of the vocal cords and the cuff has to be inflated with some air to avoid the formation of sharp edges moving forwards and backwards with respiration and causing harm to the laryngeal structures (Dillier et al. 2004). In children, inflation of the cuff to a constant pressure of 20 cmH$_2$O appears to cause minimal or no damage to the mucosa and is therefore often used (Kutter *et al.* 2013); in adults, with the main focus being the avoidance of microaspirations, slightly higher pressures, i.e. 20–30 cmH$_2$O, are recommended (Blot *et al.* 2014).

Cuffed ETTs are now well established in paediatric anaesthesia, provided that they have an adequate design (Weiss *et al.* 2004). It has been shown in a large multicentre study that they do no more side effects, e.g. stridor, than uncuffed tubes but have the advantage that changing of the ETT is only rarely needed (Weiss *et al.* 2009). And, at endoscopy, abnormalities were no more frequent in children who had previously been intubated with a cuffed ETT than in children who had never been intubated before (Weiss *et al.* 2013). Certain brands of cuffed ETTs, e.g. Microcuff, have the recommended age printed on the package. When the size of the tube is chosen according to these recommendations and the tube is inserted to the recommended depth with the ETT mark at the lower incisors, correct position is achieved in almost all patients (Weiss *et al.* 2006). This development has greatly simplified the procedure for practitioners who only occasionally treat paediatric patients.

Post-extubation croup can occur, even when a correctly sized tube is used. However, with the frequent use of dexamethasone to prevent postoperative nausea and vomiting or as co-analgesic medication, the author has the impression that post-extubation stridor has become a very rare event. On the other hand, evidence of a clear benefit of dexamethasone for the prevention of post-extubation stridor is scarce (Khemani *et al.* 2009) and almost absent for its treatment. Most practitioners, however, will rely on the knowledge gained from the treatment of infectious croup, where corticosteroids are widely recommended (Bjornson *et al.* 2004). In addition, in severe cases, inhalation of adrenaline is used, which usually provides rapid but sometimes short-lived improvement (Bjornson *et al.* 2013). Although it is widespread, the use of mist or increased humidity of the inspired gas mixture is not evidence-based.

The author has seen several cases of acquired **subglottic stenosis**; all of these patients had a history of long-term intubation, inappropriately sized ETTs and/or infection. He remembers an infant less than 1 month of age, who was ventilated with high-frequency oscillatory ventilation (HFOV) for over a week because of a severe RSV infection; because of a leak with the uncuffed size 3.5 ETT he was intubated with a size 4.0 uncuffed ETT; after a delay of a few weeks, he presented with a severe subglottic stenosis necessitating surgery (Fig. 3.5).

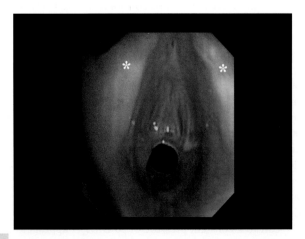

Figure 3.5 Severe subglottic stenosis after prolonged intubation in a small infant; all three factors came together: a relatively large tube, infection and mechanical damage by movements caused by HFOV (asterisks: vocal cords).

Summary and Recommendations

This case illustrates that even a short-term intubation with an inappropriately large ETT can lead to subglottic damage.

Cuffed ETTs allow successful ventilation without leak and almost eliminate the need for exchanging the ETT because of inappropriate size.

Cuffed ETTs should have an appropriate design, should be positioned with the cuff below the laryngeal structures, and should be inflated at a constant pressure of 20 cmH_2O.

References

Bjornson, C., Russell, K., Vandermeer, B., *et al.* (2013). Nebulized epinephrine for croup in children. *Cochrane Database Syst Rev*, (10), CD006619.

Bjornson, C.L., Klassen, T.P., Williamson, J., *et al.* (2004). A randomized trial of a single dose of oral dexamethasone for mild croup. *N Engl J Med*, 351, 1306–1313.

Blot, S.I., Poelaert, J., & Kollef, M. (2014). How to avoid microaspiration? A key element for the prevention of ventilator-associated pneumonia in intubated ICU patients. *BMC Infect Dis*, 14, 119.

Dillier, C.M., Trachsel, D., Baulig, W., *et al.* (2004). Laryngeal damage due to an unexpectedly large and inappropriately designed cuffed pediatric tracheal tube in a 13-month-old child. *Can J Anaesth*, 51, 72–75.

Khemani, R.G., Randolph, A., & Markovitz, B. (2009). Corticosteroids for the prevention and treatment of post-extubation stridor in neonates, children and adults. *Cochrane Database Syst Rev*, (3), CD001000.

Kutter, A.P., Bittermann, A.G., Bettschart-Wolfensberger, R., *et al.* (2013). Do lower cuff pressures reduce damage to the tracheal mucosa? A scanning electron microscopy study in neonatal pigs. *Paediatr Anaesth*, 23, 117–121.

Weiss, M., Dave, M., Bailey, M., *et al.* (2013). Endoscopic airway findings in children with or without prior endotracheal intubation. *Paediatr Anaesth*, 23, 103–110.

Weiss, M., Dullenkopf, A., & Böttcher, S. (2006). Clinical evaluation of cuff and tube tip position in a newly designed paediatric preformed oral cuffed tracheal tube. *Br J Anaesth*, 97, 695–700.

Weiss, M., Dullenkopf, A., Fischer, J.E., *et al.* (2009). Prospective randomized controlled multi-centre trial of cuffed or uncuffed endotracheal tubes in small children. *Br J Anaesth*, 103, 867–873.

Weiss, M., Dullenkopf, A., Gysin, C., *et al.* (2004). Shortcomings of cuffed paediatric tracheal tubes. *Br J Anaesth*, 92, 78–88.

3.6 Insertion Depth of the Endotracheal Tube

Case

In the early morning, an 11-year-old girl with known asthma and increasing dyspnoea felt unwell, went to the bathroom and collapsed. When her parents found her she was unresponsive and they began chest compressions. A few minutes later, the ambulance crew arrived. They performed tracheal intubation with a size 6.5 cuffed endotracheal tube (ETT) and administered adrenaline. Spontaneous circulation was restored with acceptable blood pressures. However, ventilation was extremely difficult despite the administration of ketamine and rocuronium, and the oxygen saturation remained at 60%.

The child was transferred to the children's hospital. On arrival, the 21 cm mark of the ETT was found to be at the level of the lips. The tube was pulled out by almost 4 cm. This manoeuvre was followed by a steady rise in oxygen saturation over the next few minutes to values above 90%. In the intensive care unit, asthma treatment included salbutamol by inhalation and intravenous corticosteroids. She steadily improved and could be weaned from the ventilator over the following 2 days.

Discussion

This case illustrates that the correct **insertion depth** of the ETT is of paramount importance. The correct position of the tip of the endotracheal tube should avoid endobronchial intubation in case of flexion as well as accidental extubation in case of extension of the cervical spine. Especially in the very young, the cervical spine is extremely mobile. It has been shown that the tip of the endotracheal tube can move ± 1 cm in a neonate and ± 2 cm in a 10-year-old child, caused only by movements of the cervical spine (Weiss *et al.* 2006). The length of the trachea in a term neonate is only 4 cm; for such an infant, the intended **position of the tip of the ETT** is the midpoint of the trachea, i.e. 2 cm above the carina. In a 5-year-old child it is 3 cm, and in an adolescent 4 cm above the carina. Particularly in the presence of a pneumoperitoneum, the correct ETT position is essential to avoid endobronchial intubation (Böttcher-Haberzeth *et al.* 2007).

The correct depth of insertion of the ETT can be calculated using **age-based formulas**. In neonates, the '1,2,3 kg – 7,8,9 cm rule' can be applied (Peterson *et al.* 2006): the insertion depths for oral intubation are 7, 8 and 9 cm for a 1 kg, 2 kg and 3 kg baby, respectively. For nasotracheal intubation, 20% has to be added. From the age of 1 year, using the formula **12 cm + ½ cm per year** results in good estimates for ETT insertion depth for oral intubation. In our patient, an insertion depth of 12 cm + 11/2 cm = 17.5 cm could be expected, and 21 cm was far too deep. In adults, oral ETT insertion depths of 20 cm for women and 22 cm for men may be appropriate (Roberts *et al.* 1995, Sitzwohl *et al.* 2010). It is part of good practice to

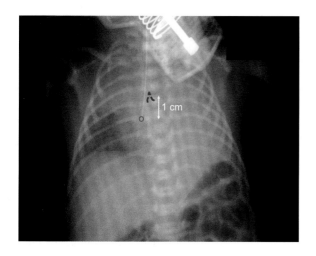

Figure 3.6 A chest x-ray of a 2 kg preterm neonate who was intubated in respiratory distress for surfactant administration. The nasotracheal tube was inserted 12 cm instead of the expected 9.6 cm, leading to atelectasis of the left lung and the right upper lobe.

know the approximate ETT insertion depth before we approach the child. Of course, the passage of the ETT between the cords is observed until the markings on the tube are in the correct position. This is ultimately more reliable than the age-based formulas (Weiss *et al.* 2005). Up to school age, the passage of the tip of the ETT can be palpated very easily in the cervical trachea (Bednarek & Kuhns 1975); a suprasternal position just at the jugulum is optimal (Jain *et al.* 2004). Deliberate main-stem intubation and auscultation while the tube is withdrawn until bilateral equal breath sounds are heard is nowadays only rarely used (Mariano *et al.* 2005). Equal breath sounds heard over both lungs do not rule out endobronchial intubation, especially when ETTs with a Murphy eye are used (Verghese *et al.* 2004). In case of any uncertainty, fibreoptic verification of the correct ETT position is recommended.

In **individuals with healthy lungs** even deep endobronchial intubation results in atelectasis formation in the non-ventilated areas, with decreased tidal volumes or higher than usual peak pressures. In the short term, e.g. intraoperatively, life-threatening desaturations rarely occur when higher concentrations of inspired oxygen are used. Problems often arise after surgery, when the extubated child now presents with respiratory failure requiring re-intubation. In contrast, in patients with pre-existing lung disease, such as a severe asthma attack with ventilation/perfusion mismatch, as in this case, profound life-threatening hypoxaemia will develop.

This story of an **asthmatic child** also shows that even when a diagnosis is known, the initiation of therapy may be delayed unnecessarily in emergency situations. Beta-2-agonists by inhalation are usually highly effective; in addition, intravenous corticosteroids should be given early.

Summary and Recommendations

This case highlights the importance of correct ETT insertion depth. Age-based formulas should be used to estimate the appropriate depth before the patient is approached.

In patients with sick lungs, an endobronchial intubation can cause a 'can intubate, cannot ventilate' situation and lead to fatalities.

The timely treatment of the underlying disease, in this case asthma, should not be delayed after the initial steps of resuscitation or on transport.

References

Bednarek, F.J. & Kuhns, L.R. (1975). Endotracheal tube placement in infants determined by suprasternal palpation: a new technique. *Pediatrics*, 56, 224–229.

Böttcher-Haberzeth, S., Dullenkopf, A., Gitzelmann, C.A., *et al.* (2007). Tracheal tube tip displacement during laparoscopy in children. *Anaesthesia*, 62, 131–134.

Jain, A., Finer, N.N., Hilton, S., *et al.* (2004). A randomized trial of suprasternal palpation to determine endotracheal tube position in neonates. *Resuscitation*, 60, 297–302.

Mariano, E.R., Ramamoorthy, C., Chu, L.F., *et al.* (2005). A comparison of three methods for estimating appropriate tracheal tube depth in children. *Paediatr Anaesth*, 15, 846–885.

Peterson, J., Johnson, N., Deakins, K., *et al.* (2006). Accuracy of the 7-8-9 Rule for endotracheal tube placement in the neonate. *J Perinatol*, 26, 333–336.

Roberts, J.R., Spadafora, M., & Cone, D.C. (1995). Proper depth placement of oral endotracheal tubes in adults prior to radiographic confirmation. *Acad Emerg Med*, 2, 20–24.

Sitzwohl, C., Langheinrich, A., Schober, A., *et al.* (2010). Endobronchial intubation detected by insertion depth of endotracheal tube, bilateral auscultation, or observation of chest movements: randomised trial. *BMJ*, 341, c5943.

Verghese, S.T., Hannallah, R.S., Slack, M.C., *et al.* (2004). Auscultation of bilateral breath sounds does not rule out endobronchial intubation in children. *Anesth Analg*, 99, 56–58.

Weiss, M., Balmer, C., Dullenkopf, A., *et al.* (2005). Intubation depth markings allow an improved positioning of endotracheal tubes in children. *Can J Anaesth*, 52, 721–726.

Weiss, M., Knirsch, W., Kretschmar, O., *et al.* (2006). Tracheal tube tip displacement in children during head-neck movement: a radiological assessment. *Br J Anaesth*, 96, 486–491.

Case 3.7

Laryngeal Perforation

Case

At 19 weeks of gestation, a fetus presented with a large neck mass, which gradually increased over the following weeks. It obviously impeded fetal swallowing, leading to massive polyhydramnios requiring repeated amniocentesis.

An EXIT (ex utero intrapartum treatment) procedure was proposed but declined by the mother. Therefore, an elective caesarean section was meticulously planned and performed under optimal conditions at 33 weeks of gestation in an operating room at the children's hospital. In addition to a senior anaesthetist and a senior neonatologist, an ENT and a paediatric surgeon, both fully equipped, were present in the room. The time point was chosen because of poorly controllable polyhydramnios.

After delivery, the baby presented with minimal muscle tone and absent respiratory effort. Without delay, direct laryngoscopy with a Miller blade size 1 was performed. Surprisingly, the vocal cords could easily be visualized and intubation with an endotracheal tube (ETT) size 3.0 with an inserted but non-protruding stylet was attempted. After passing the vocal cords, resistance was encountered. After administering a slight, but not unusual pressure, a sudden give was felt and a yellow watery fluid, followed by blood, flooded the field. Ventilation was attempted but resulted in only minimal movements of the neck mass (Fig. 3.7). Repeated laryngoscopy confirmed that the ETT had passed the vocal cords, but when the ENT specialist performed rigid bronchoscopy, only a dark black region beyond the cords could be seen. After 30 minutes of unsuccessful resuscitation efforts, the baby was declared dead.

Post-mortem examination showed a teratoma weighing 340 g. After dissection from the tumour, the trachea appeared normal with no signs of obstruction. However, there was a large, longitudinal 4 mm perforation at the level of the cricothyroid membrane.

Discussion

In this patient with a **giant neck mass**, difficult intubation owing to a distorted, compressed or even completely obstructed airway was anticipated. Surprisingly, this was not the case and laryngoscopy was performed without difficulty. At autopsy, after dissection of the teratoma, the trachea was anatomically normal. Probably, face-mask ventilation or ventilation by a laryngeal mask airway (LMA) would have been possible, even though there was massive distortion of the trachea. A final attempt of face-mask ventilation has been recommended in recent guidelines for adults before proceeding to a surgical airway (Frerk *et al.* 2015). In the case described here, mask ventilation was never tried because the primary goal for the team was to rapidly secure the potentially completely compressed airway with

47

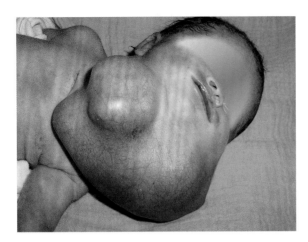

Figure 3.7 The large cervical teratoma did not impede direct laryngoscopy, but the insertion of the ETT led to laryngeal perforation.

an ETT without losing precious time. Following injury of the cricothyroid membrane, face-mask ventilation would probably have resulted in subcutaneous emphysema.

But, unexpectedly, another airway complication occurred when **the cricothyroid membrane was perforated** by the tip of the ETT. During endotracheal intubation, the tip of the ETT comes in contact with the cricothyroid membrane and can cause damage. This is especially true for very small babies, because the tissue is very fragile (Berger & Fontana 2010). In the presented case, the laryngeal structures were fixed by surrounding abnormal tissue completely eliminating the mobility of the cervical trachea and the laryngeal structures, which usually prevents injury when pressure is applied. Several long-serving paediatric anaesthetists have experienced similar catastrophic events, which are likely to be under-reported in the anaesthetic and paediatric literature (Wei & Bond 2011). Ventilation through an ETT positioned within the soft tissues of the neck will rapidly lead to subcutaneous emphysema, bilateral pneumothorax and fatal outcome (Berger & Fontana 2010, Doherty *et al.* 2005).

Therefore, the prevention of any type of **airway trauma** is of paramount importance. During nasotracheal intubation the ETT approaches the larynx from a posterior position in an anterior direction and meets the cricothyroid membrane almost perpendicularly. The ETT should never be moved forcefully in this direction by using a Magill forceps. The tip of the ETT should only be placed between the vocal cords and then advanced manually under slight rotation, perhaps even supported by some inclination of the cervical spine, which leads to a better alignment of the trachea and the ETT. An even more gentle approach might be to first advance a thin suction catheter through the ETT into the trachea, and then to railroad the tube over it (Berger & Fontana 2010). During orotracheal intubation, it is wise to avoid the use of a stylet in all but a few exceptional cases. A stylet should never protrude beyond the tip of the ETT. Finally, force must never be applied.

Even if an **EXIT procedure** had been performed in this case, a similar airway trauma could have resulted. The principle of the EXIT procedure is to perform a caesarean section and to first deliver just the head and one shoulder and arm of the baby (to allow pulse oximetry monitoring), while the placental circulation remains intact and continues to provide gas exchange (Hartnick *et al.* 2009). The medical team thus has time to find a solution for a congenital upper airway obstruction. Periods of up to 60 minutes on placental circulation during an EXIT procedure have been reported (Lazar *et al.* 2011). For the procedure, profound uterine relaxation is required, which, coupled with a prolonged period from uterine incision to uterine repair, puts the pregnant women at a significant risk for bleeding complications. This is why the mother in this case declined an EXIT procedure.

Summary and Recommendations

The laryngeal structures are vulnerable, and perforation of the cricothyroid membrane can occur, especially if the patient is very small or if the laryngeal structures are surrounded by tissue impeding the normal high mobility of the cervical trachea.

Every precaution should be taken to avoid airway trauma. During nasotracheal intubation, the Magill forceps should not be used to push the ETT into the trachea, but only to place it on top of the posterior commissure between the arytenoids; from there it should be advanced gently under slight rotation into the trachea.

This case also illustrates that a trial of face-mask ventilation is reasonable when everything else fails, before proceeding to an anterior neck approach or even discontinuing resuscitation.

References

Berger, T.M. & Fontana, M. (2010). Fatal tracheal rupture in an extremely preterm infant. Case of the month, October 2010. Swiss Society of Neonatology. www.neonet.ch/files/9314/2591/5116/COTM_october_2010.pdf (accessed 29 November 2017).

Doherty, K.M., Tabaee, A., Castillo, M., *et al.* (2005). Neonatal tracheal rupture complicating endotracheal intubation: a case report and indications for conservative management. *Int J Pediatr Otorhinolaryngol*, 69, 111–116.

Frerk, C., Mitchell, V.S., McNarry, A.F., *et al.* (2015). Difficult Airway Society 2015 guidelines for management of unanticipated difficult intubation in adults. *Br J Anaesth*, 115, 827–848.

Hartnick, C.J., Barth, W.H., Coté, C.J., *et al.* (2009). Case records of the Massachusetts General Hospital. Case 7-2009. A pregnant woman with a large mass in the fetal oral cavity. *N Engl J Med*, 360, 913–921.

Lazar, D.A., Olutoye, O.O., Moise, K.J., *et al.* (2011). Ex-utero intrapartum treatment procedure for giant neck masses: fetal and maternal outcomes. *J Pediatr Surg*, 46, 817–822.

Wei, J.L. & Bond, J. (2011). Management and prevention of endotracheal intubation injury in neonates. *Curr Opin Otolaryngol Head Neck Surg*, 19, 474–477.

Bronchial Rupture

Case

One late afternoon, a 12-year-old boy, weighing 60 kg, was hit by a car. He was found on the scene with a Glasgow Coma Scale (GCS) score of 3 and a bleeding facial laceration. He was intubated by an emergency physician with a size 8.0 cuffed endotracheal tube (ETT) down to an insertion depth of 24 cm, and then transported to the children's hospital. On arrival, diminished breath sounds over the left lung were identified, suggesting endobronchial intubation, and the ETT was withdrawn by 3 cm. On chest x-ray, a pneumomediastinum, as well as subcutaneous and intra-abdominal air, was identified (Fig. 3.8). The pupils were small and reactive and a cranial CT scan showed no major lesions. Clinically, a subcutaneous emphysema extending down to the scrotum and a distended abdomen became increasingly obvious.

He was taken to theatre for the insertion of a chest drain and an intracranial pressure-monitoring device. When the subcutaneous emphysema continued to increase and a massive air leak via the chest drain was noted, fibreoptic bronchoscopy was performed. The examination revealed a laceration of the posterior tracheal wall with a length of 3 cm, extending from the tip of the ETT down to the carina. The cardiothoracic and ENT surgeons were called for advice, and surgical repair via right thoracotomy was planned. Intubation of the left main bronchus under fibreoptic guidance with a size 7.0 cuffed reinforced ETT did not allow sufficient ventilation despite the use of high ventilation pressures. Therefore the ETT was withdrawn to a tracheal position, resulting in adequate gas exchange. During surgical repair, which also involved the use of a pericardial flap, the cuff of the ETT was deflated and a Cook airway exchange catheter was placed through the ETT into the right main bronchus. This device was used for manual jet ventilation over 90 minutes. The patient was extubated on postoperative day 3 and made an uneventful recovery.

Discussion

This case of a **tracheal rupture** following blunt thoracic trauma and endotracheal intubation illustrates that early bronchoscopy is mandatory when a massive air leak via a chest drain is noted (Fig. 3.8). The case has already been reported in part elsewhere (Ruppen *et al.* 2002). The exact origin of the tracheal tear in this case remains unknown. Blunt chest trauma with acute massive forward flexion can lead to rupture of the tracheobronchial tree with a longitudinal tear in the membranous part of the trachea, typically located close to the carina or even extending into the right main-stem bronchus. On the other hand, iatrogenic damage by a protruding stylet, or probably more frequently by overinflating the cuff, are quite common and can cause a similar picture (Paraschiv 2014).

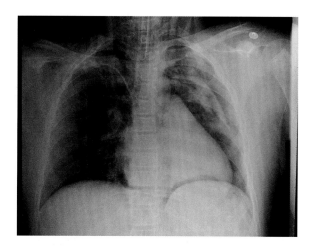

Figure 3.8 Chest x-ray of a 12-year-old child with tracheal rupture and massive air leak syndrome with pneumomediastinum and subcutaneous emphysema.

The **treatment modalities** in case of bronchial rupture vary. When the lesion can easily be bridged with an ETT, conservative management can be an excellent option (Frova & Sorbello 2011). Otherwise, surgical repair is the preferred option. Airway management during surgical repair is challenging, and close cooperation with the surgeon is very important. The use of a double-lumen ETT is often not an ideal option because of the risk of additional trauma during the insertion and because its fixed position often interferes with surgery. The author has personally used endobronchial intubation (Besmer *et al.* 2001) and, in two cases, manual jet ventilation via a venous catheter or (as in the presented case) a Cook airway-exchange catheter (Ruppen *et al.* 2002). The surgeon can guide these devices into the desired position in the main bronchus.

Manual jet ventilation is a rescue technique that was not originally designed for prolonged ventilation. The anaesthetist has to be very careful, because pressures and volumes cannot be measured precisely. In addition, airway occlusion caused by extremely dry secretions is a continuous threat since these devices are typically used without a humidification system. In the future, use of the Ventrain system, which also supports expiration and therefore helps to avoid lung overdistension, will probably replace the classic manual jet ventilation (Willemsen *et al.* 2014).

The presented case also illustrates that manipulation of an ETT can lead to dramatic changes. When the ETT was withdrawn by 3 cm, the subcutaneous emphysema increased rapidly, probably because the tip of the ETT was moved into a position above the tracheal tear. Rarely, a mistake, such as advancing an ETT too far, can by chance be beneficial or even life-saving (Besmer *et al.* 2001).

Summary and Recommendations

The presented case illustrates that in the presence of a massive air leak or progressive subcutaneous emphysema, bronchial rupture should be considered and early bronchoscopy is mandatory.

Management of a bronchial tear is very challenging, and the anaesthetist has to be very versatile to find the best technique for airway management, adapted to the individual case.

Manipulation of an ETT can lead to unexpected events, and close observation of the patient following any adjustments is important.

References

Besmer, I., Schüpfer, G., Stulz, P., *et al.* (2001). Tracheal rupture: delayed diagnosis with endobronchial intubation [in German]. *Anaesthesist*, 50, 167–170.

Frova, G. & Sorbello, M. (2011). Iatrogenic tracheobronchial ruptures: the debate continues. *Minerva Anestesiol*, 77, 1130–1133.

Paraschiv, M. (2014). Iatrogenic tracheobronchial rupture. *J Med Life*, 7, 343–348.

Ruppen, W., Schlegel, C., Kistler, W., *et al.* (2002). Tracheal rupture in a 12 year-old-child: a possible complication of tracheal intubation? *Paediatr Anaesth*, 12, 465–466.

Willemsen, M.G., Noppens, R., Mulder, A.L., *et al.* (2014). Ventilation with the Ventrain through a small lumen catheter in the failed paediatric airway: two case reports. *Br J Anaesth*, 112, 946–947.

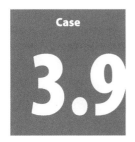

Damage to Teeth

Case

A 3-year-old girl, weighing 14 kg, was scheduled for inguinal hernia repair. After premedication with 12 mg (0.86 mg/kg) of rectal midazolam, anaesthesia was induced by mask with sevoflurane and nitrous oxide; a classic type laryngeal mask airway (LMA) was inserted using the rotational technique and a caudal block was performed in a left lateral position. While the patient was being turned back to a supine position, traces of blood were seen in the mouth and a broken front tooth was noticed. The dentition was partly destroyed by caries. The decision was made to proceed with surgery and to ask the maxillofacial surgeon for a second opinion at the end of the case.

The specialist advised removing the residual dental root in order to prevent infection and pain. The parents waiting on the ward were informed and gave consent for the residual dental root to be removed. The girl made an uneventful recovery; she was later referred for further treatment of the extensively carious primary dentition under general anaesthesia.

Discussion

It is very likely that only slight pressure by the LMA during positioning for the caudal block was sufficient to fracture the already very fragile carious tooth in this case. Normally, in contrast to adults, where the approximate incidence may be 1:5000 anaesthetics (Nouette-Gaulain *et al.* 2012, Warner *et al.* 1999), **damage to teeth** is not a common topic in paediatric anaesthesia textbooks. Most do not even mention this complication, because neonates and young infants have no visible teeth, the primary teeth are small, mouth opening is wide and the secondary teeth are initially healthy and very robust in young adolescents.

However, the unerupted tooth buds can be injured by pressure of the laryngoscope on the gums even in **preterm babies**. This can lead to abnormal dental development, maleruption and enamel hypoplasia, typically of the upper right incisor (Noren *et al.* 1993, Suely Falcao de Oliveira Melo *et al.* 2014). It is very likely that even irreversible damage to dentition can be caused by neonatal intubation (Seow *et al.* 1990). As these complications are only seen years after a traumatic intubation, anaesthetists and neonatologists usually do not become aware of them.

The **primary dentition** begins to erupt by the age of 6 months and is usually complete by 2 years of age. As the permanent teeth erupt, the roots of the primary teeth are resorbed; the deciduous teeth lose their alveolar support and are finally kept in place only by ligamentous structures. At this stage, only slight force can make them mobile. The author is aware of a mother who was extremely upset because, after an uneventful anaesthetic, her

(a)

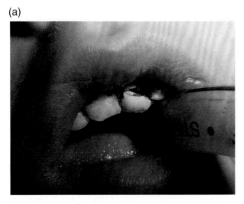

(b)

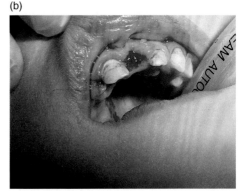

Figure 3.9a A fractured carious tooth.

Figure 3.9b The maxillofacial surgeon removed the fractured dental root, and thus the problem was fixed during the current anaesthetic.

6-year-old daughter reported that she now also had a mobile maxillary anterior tooth. Children should be asked if they have loose teeth, because visual inspection will show normal teeth and not necessarily identify any mobility.

Quite often parents request the removal of a very **loose deciduous tooth** while their child is under general anaesthesia. While the risk of accidental loss and aspiration of a loose tooth during anaesthesia should be taken into account, they should not routinely be removed during the natural process of resorption of the root of the primary tooth and eruption of the second dentition.

In the presented case, **massive caries** was the main causative factor for the fracture of the tooth. In everyday life, biting on hard food particles could have led to an identical result (Fig. 3.9a). However, the fact is that the child came with a carious but still functional tooth and left without it; the open dental pulp of the fractured root could have resulted in infection and pain within hours or days. To minimize suffering for the patient, an appropriate decision was made to delay the list, not to wake up the child and send her to the dentist for later removal of the root, but to use the hospital's facilities, to call the maxillofacial surgeon and to have the problem fixed during the current anaesthetic (Fig. 3.9b).

Abnormal dentition (dentinogenesis imperfecta) typically occurs with **osteogenesis imperfecta** (Malmgren & Norgren 2002). Therefore, the anaesthetist should be aware not only of the increased fragility of the osseous structures in such patients, but also of the vulnerability of their teeth.

It is all about **prevention**. In most cases, damage to teeth can be avoided when abnormal fragility of the dentition is recognized in advance. In such a case, avoidance of any airway instrumentation and reliance on intravenous sedation and regional anaesthesia is an attractive alternative. If an LMA is used, special care is needed at the time of insertion and, even more importantly, at the time of removal. Any agitation while the airway is still in place has to be avoided. It is the author's practice to remove the airway in such cases in the deeply anaesthetized spontaneously breathing child. Of course, laryngoscopy is the most risky manoeuvre. In adults, preference is frequently given to awake fibreoptic intubation to avoid any oral manipulation, but this is rarely an option in children.

Summary and Recommendations

Damage to teeth can also occur in children, especially when carious dentition is present.

In neonates, the unerupted tooth can be damaged by pressure caused by the laryngoscope; skilled and atraumatic intubation is mandatory.

If fragile teeth are recognized in time, further injury can usually be avoided.

References

Malmgren, B. & Norgren, S. (2002). Dental aberrations in children and adolescents with osteogenesis imperfecta. *Acta Odontol Scand*, 60, 65–71.

Noren, J.G., Ranggard, L., Klingberg, G., Persson, C., & Nilsson, K. (1993). Intubation and mineralization disturbances in the enamel of primary teeth. *Acta Odontol Scand*, 51, 271–275.

Nouette-Gaulain, K., Lenfant, F., Jacquet-Francillon, D., *et al.* (2012). French clinical guidelines for prevention of perianaesthetic dental injuries: long text [in French]. *Ann Fr Anesth Reanim*, 31, 213–223.

Seow, W.K., Perham, S., Young, W.G., *et al.* (1990). Dilaceration of a primary maxillary incisor associated with neonatal laryngoscopy. *Pediatr Dent*, 12, 321–324.

Suely Falcao de Oliveira Melo, N., Guimaraes Vieira Cavalcante da Silva, R.P., & Adilson Soares de Lima, A. (2014). The neonatal intubation causes defects in primary teeth of premature infants. *Biomed Pap Med Fac Univ Palacky Olomouc Czech Repub*, 158, 605–612.

Warner, M.E., Benenfeld, S.M., Warner, M.A., *et al.* (1999). Perianesthetic dental injuries: frequency, outcomes, and risk factors. *Anesthesiology*, 90, 1302–1305.

3.10

Damage Related to a Supraglottic Airway

Case

An 11-year-old boy, weighing 50 kg, was scheduled for circumcision under general anaesthesia combined with a penile block. Anaesthesia was induced by mask with sevoflurane and nitrous oxide and a classic type laryngeal mask airway (LMA) size 3 was inserted using the rotational technique. Because of an apparent leakage it was replaced with an LMA of the same type, but now size 4. Anaesthesia was switched to an intravenous technique with propofol and remifentanil and a penile block was performed. Nitrous oxide was no longer used for maintenance. The further anaesthetic course was uneventful. The patient also received ondansetron 4 mg (0.08 mg/kg), dexamethasone 8 mg (0.16 mg/kg) and ketorolac 30 mg (0.6 mg/kg).

One hour after the end of surgery, the anaesthetist was called to the day surgery unit because the patient complained about numbness of the tongue, predominantly on the left side. The patient was informed that this could be related to the used airway device, that the phenomenon was harmless and that the symptoms would disappear spontaneously over the next few hours or days. The patient was followed up by telephone, and on postoperative day 5 the sensibility of the tongue was reported to be normal again.

Discussion

The described symptoms correspond to a **lingual nerve neurapraxia**, the most common nerve injury associated with the use of a supraglottic airway device. More frequent morbidities following the use of an LMA are sore throat, minor mucosal abrasions, dysphagia and occasional hoarseness; **cranial nerve injury**, on the other hand, is a rare event (Thiruvenkatarajan et al. 2015). The lingual nerve, a pure sensory branch of the mandibular nerve, is most commonly affected. It runs along the mandible directly under the mucosa and can be compressed or stretched by the cuff of the LMA. Usually, there is spontaneous recovery within hours or days; however, in the meantime, the loss of sensation and taste as well as impaired speech and the risk of tongue injury can significantly disturb the patient. It is important that anaesthetists are familiar with the condition and are able to reassure the parents and the child. Although only around two dozen cases have been reported in the literature (Thiruvenkatarajan et al. 2015), the true incidence of transient lingual nerve apraxia following the use of an LMA is probably much higher and in part dependent on close and complete follow-up. The author remembers three children, in all of them the symptoms disappeared after one week at the latest.

The **hypoglossal nerve** is also vulnerable to compression by an overinflated or malpositioned LMA cuff. It is a pure motor nerve, and paresis leads to dysphagia and dysarthria.

Because of their anatomical proximity, the hypoglossal and lingual nerves are sometimes simultaneously affected. Patients with hypoglossal nerve paralysis should be seen by a neurologist, because other causes (e.g. carotid artery dissection) are possible, and recovery usually takes longer. The most relevant neurological complication associated with LMA use is **recurrent laryngeal nerve damage**, which frequently presents with significant morbidity (Endo *et al.* 2007). Unilateral paresis will cause hoarseness and an elevated risk of aspiration; bilateral paresis may even necessitate tracheotomy. Fortunately, barely more than a dozen cases have been reported in the literature.

Nerve injury has been reported with most of the commonly used classic type, Pro-Seal and Supreme LMAs. However, it has also been described with the use of the I-Gel device (Theron & Loyden 2008), which indicates that overinflation of the cuff (e.g. by diffusion of nitrous oxide) is not the only factor contributing to nerve injury.

Several factors contribute to LMA-associated nerve injuries, and even when the device is used with a proper technique they may not be completely preventable. The selection of the appropriate **size** of the supraglottic airway device is of paramount importance. Most manufactures recommend weight-based selection of the device, but other aspects should also be considered, including gender, oropharyngeal dimensions or laryngeal growth during male puberty. Often, the decision is made based on a feeling guided by experience. For the classic type, and the Pro-Seal, the size of the external ear has been proposed as a guide to size selection (Haliloglu *et al.* 2017). In the author's opinion, extreme rotation of the head, e.g. for bat ear surgery, may be harmful too.

It is very likely that a size 4 classic type LMA was rather large for the 11-year-old boy in this case, although he had reached the weight limit of 50 kg. In addition, the airway device should be in an **optimal position** in order to avoid the need for overinflating the cuff for a good seal. The **cuff pressure** should be measured and adjusted to less than 60 cmH$_2$O (von Ungern-Sternberg *et al.* 2009) or perhaps even less than 40 cmH$_2$O (Jagannathan *et al.* 2013). If nitrous oxide is used for maintenance, its diffusion into the cuff has to be considered (Maino *et al.* 2005).

Summary and Recommendations

This is a typical case of lingual nerve neurapraxia following the use of a rather generously sized LMA.

An adequately sized and optimally positioned supraglottic airway device may help to prevent this complication.

LMA cuff pressure must be measured and limited to less than 40–60 cmH$_2$O.

References

Endo, K., Okabe, Y., Maruyama, Y., *et al.* (2007). Bilateral vocal cord paralysis caused by laryngeal mask airway. *Am J Otolaryngol*, 28, 126–129.

Haliloglu, M., Bilgen, S., Uzture, N., *et al.* (2017). Simple method for determining the size of the ProSeal laryngeal mask airway in children: a prospective observational study. *Braz J Anesthesiol*, 67, 15–20.

Jagannathan, N., Sohn, L., Sommers, K., *et al.* (2013). A randomized comparison of the laryngeal mask airway supreme and laryngeal mask airway unique in infants and children: does cuff pressure influence leak pressure? *Paediatr Anaesth*, 23, 927–933.

Maino, P., Dullenkopf, A., Bernet, V., *et al.* (2005). Nitrous oxide diffusion into the cuffs of disposable laryngeal mask airways. *Anaesthesia*, 60, 278–282.

Theron, A.D. & Loyden, C. (2008). Nerve damage following the use of an i-gel supraglottic airway device. *Anaesthesia*, 63, 441–442.

Thiruvenkatarajan, V., Van Wijk, R.M., & Rajbhoj, A. (2015). Cranial nerve injuries with supraglottic airway devices: a systematic review of published case reports and series. *Anaesthesia*, 70, 344–359.

von Ungern-Sternberg, B.S., Erb, T.O., Chambers, N.A., *et al.* (2009). Laryngeal mask airways: to inflate or to deflate after insertion? *Paediatr Anaesth*, 19, 837–843.

Regurgitation during the Use of a Supraglottic Airway

Case

Many years ago, an almost 4-year-old boy, weighing 17 kg, was scheduled for hypospadias repair. After inhalational induction, the airway was secured with a size 2.0 ProSeal laryngeal mask airway (LMA), and a gastric tube was inserted through the oesophageal access and left open to air. A penile block, using bupivacaine 0.75%, combined with a caudal block, using ropivacaine 0.2% and 30 μg clonidine, provided analgesia. Throughout the case, the child was breathing spontaneously a mixture of air, oxygen and 2% sevoflurane.

Surgery proceeded and the anaesthetic course was perfectly stable. After almost 3 hours, the surgeon wanted to proceed to the retrieval of oral mucosa needed for urethral reconstruction. The tape fixing the LMA was removed and the tubing was pushed a little to one side to achieve good surgical exposure. Suddenly, the child was bucking and ventilation stopped. A brownish fluid came out of the gastric tube, but was also seen in the ventilator tubing. Oxygen saturation started to decline, and the anaesthetist called for help.

Thiopental and mivacurium were given, and the sevoflurane concentration was increased. The gastric tube as well as the lumen of the LMA were suctioned to remove the brownish secretions. Ventilation was now controlled and a PEEP of 5 cmH_2O was applied according to routine practice. Fibreoptic inspection showed brownish secretions at the level of the LMA and copious secretions in the bronchial tree, but no particulate material. Initially, elevated inspiratory pressures and an FiO_2 of at least 50% were needed to maintain saturation above 93%. Fortunately, by the end of the case, the child was breathing spontaneously with an FiO_2 of 30% and the LMA was removed (Fig. 3.11). The further course was uneventful.

Discussion

The presented case of **regurgitation** and aspiration in a spontaneously breathing child with an LMA in place serves to highlight several educational points.

First, the **LMA protects the airway** perfectly against blood and secretions coming from above, e.g. during tonsillectomy. However, aspiration of gastric content is still possible. In a review of the literature, 23 cases were identified, including six children (Keller *et al.* 2004a). In the majority of these cases, predisposing or avoidable factors were described. The gastric access ports of the second-generation devices, including among others ProSeal, Supreme and AuraGain, do not preclude aspiration. Theoretically, regurgitated material should bypass the pharynx, as has been reported in adults (Mark 2003) and in children (Keller *et al.* 2004b). However, when a large amount of fluid is expelled under high pressure, some material can still enter the larynx, as illustrated by the present case. It is noteworthy that a

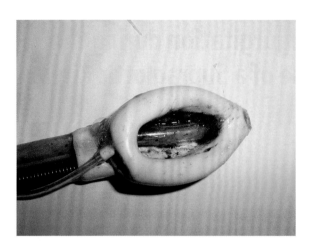

Figure 3.11 This ProSeal LMA did not protect against regurgitation and aspiration of gastric content.

paediatric 10F gastric tube, which fits in a size 2 LMA, almost completely obstructs the lumen of the gastric access, and the resistance of the gastric tube itself is very high. The benefits of the second-generation device may thus be lost, as it now behaves like a classic type LMA.

Second, sufficient **depth of anaesthesia** is a prerequisite for a safe and smooth anaesthetic course. Spontaneous regurgitation is a rare event during anaesthesia (el Mikatti *et al.* 1995). In most cases, regurgitation, vomiting and aspiration are provoked by manipulations during planes of anaesthesia that are too light (Lussmann & Gerber 1997). Surgery was perfectly tolerated in the genital region because of the concomitant effects of regional anaesthesia, but as soon as the surgeon began to work in the oral cavity, an arousal reaction with increased intra-abdominal pressure was provoked. No doubt, better anticipation could have prevented this complication by increasing sevoflurane and administering an opioid or perhaps, even better, neuromuscular blockade. In this case a BIS monitor had been used, showing values in the 30s before the event, but EEG-based monitors primarily indicate the degree of hypnosis and not the depth of anaesthesia, and therefore cannot predict what will happen after a painful stimulation. It was the author's practice to provide neuromuscular blockade whenever an LMA was used in potentially critical situations, e.g. during prolonged surgery with prone positioning or when the anaesthetist was positioned away from the head with no chance of getting to the airway.

Third, **experienced practitioners** pay attention to every detail and do not just choose the correct airway device. Endotracheal intubation would have avoided the described complication a priori, but the same could have been achieved with a sufficient depth of anaesthesia. The problem was not that an LMA was chosen for this type of procedure, but the inadequate performance of the anaesthetist. Placing a gastric tube helps to stabilize the LMA in the right place, comparable to the use of the guidewire in the Seldinger technique: the LMA will always railroad into the correct position. In addition, the gastric tube allows active evacuation of the stomach. Nevertheless, in routine cases, it is probably safer to remove the gastric tube to guarantee low-resistance outflow from the oesophagus.

Fourth, **in case of suspected regurgitation**, it is reasonable to leave the LMA in place, to suction it, and to make sure that the residual gastric content is minimal. There is no need to rush to intubation in every case.

Summary and Recommendations

The presented case illustrates that regurgitation and aspiration can occur even with a second-generation LMA.

Insufficient depth of anaesthesia, i.e. inadequate performance by the anaesthetist, is usually the basis for regurgitation and aspiration.

The use of EEG-based monitoring assures us that the patient is currently unconscious, but it does not guarantee that the patient will not react to a painful stimulus.

References

el Mikatti, N., Luthra, A.D., Healy, T.E., *et al.* (1995). Gastric regurgitation during general anaesthesia in different positions with the laryngeal mask airway. *Anaesthesia*, 50, 1053–1055.

Keller, C., Brimacombe, J., Bittersohl, J., *et al.* (2004a). Aspiration and the laryngeal mask airway: three cases and a review of the literature. *Br J Anaesth*, 93, 579–582.

Keller, C., Brimacombe, J., von Goedecke, A., *et al.* (2004b). Airway protection with the ProSeal laryngeal mask airway in a child. *Paediatr Anaesth*, 14,1021–1022.

Lussmann, R.F. & Gerber, H.R. (1997). Severe aspiration pneumonia with the laryngeal mask [in German]. *Anasthesiol Intensivmed Notfallmed Schmerzther*, 32, 194–196.

Mark, D.A. (2003). Protection from aspiration with the LMA-ProSeal after vomiting: a case report. *Can J Anaesth*, 50, 78–80.

Case 3.12 Pneumothorax

Case

Many decades ago, a 2700 g term neonate was scheduled for emergency gastroschisis repair. A peripheral intravenous line was in place, and the anaesthetic regimen included a high-dose opioid, 50 µg/kg of fentanyl as an infusion over 10 minutes preceded by pancuronium 0.15 mg/kg. An arterial catheter was inserted into the right radial artery. The event took place a long time before the arrival of ultrasound into paediatric anaesthesia practice, and several attempts to cannulate the right internal jugular vein using a 22G steel needle and the Seldinger technique failed, as did a subclavian approach. Blood could be aspirated repeatedly, but the guidewire could not be advanced without meeting resistance. Together with the surgeon, the decision was taken to proceed with surgery using peripheral venous access and to insert a Broviac catheter at the end of the case for parenteral nutrition.

During positioning for surgery, the oxygen saturation signal was lost, the blood pressure tracing showed a dampened signal, the baby turned blue and the airway pressure peaked at more than 30 cmH$_2$O. No breath sounds could be heard over the right lung. Transillumination with the surgical cold light confirmed the diagnosis of a pneumothorax. A chest drain was inserted, air escaped under pressure with a whizzing noise, and surgery proceeded as planned.

Discussion

This case of a **tension pneumothorax** in a neonate after failed central venous puncture illustrates that damage to the lungs is an ever-present threat when performing punctures at the level of the thorax or the neck. Nowadays, with the use of ultrasound, the risk of causing a pneumothorax should be minimal with the internal jugular approach, and much lower when compared to the landmark-based subclavian approach. During his professional career, the author has witnessed several cases of pneumothorax after subclavian vein catheterization (Fig. 3.12), but only a few after internal jugular vein puncture. This observation has not been confirmed in a meta-analysis of the published adult literature (Ruesch *et al.* 2002). With respect to infectious complications, the subclavian approach seems to be advantageous in children (Breschan *et al.* 2007, Camkiran *et al.* 2016), and the insertion site is undoubtedly easier to care for. A disadvantage is the much higher incidence of catheter malposition (Camkiran *et al.* 2016).

Diagnosis of a pneumothorax is classically based on a chest x-ray, although ultrasound examination is potentially faster and more sensitive (Cattarossi *et al.* 2016, Liu *et al.* 2017). For decades, transillumination has been the favoured method for rapid bedside diagnosis of

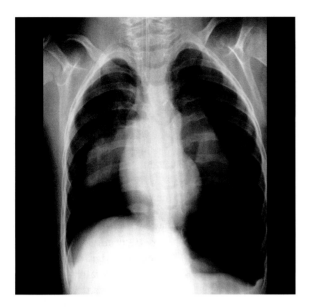

Figure 3.12 Bilateral pneumothorax after attempted subclavian vein catheterization (different patient). It is strongly recommended to avoid bilateral attempts.

a large pneumothorax in neonatology (Kuhns *et al.* 1975). Clinically, diminished breath sounds will be heard over the affected lung. In tension pneumothorax, the heart sounds are shifted to the non-affected contralateral side.

Pneumothorax may occur spontaneously in term and preterm neonates, but more often it occurs in the context of mechanical ventilation or significant lung disease, especially following meconium aspiration. In a spontaneously occurring pneumothorax in neonates, needle aspiration is often used for first-line **treatment** (Bruschettini *et al.* 2016); however, in the context of anaesthesia and surgery, intercostal tube drainage is the usual practice.

Given the inherent risk associated with venous puncture attempts in the upper part of the body, it has been the author's practice to prefer a femoral approach for short-term use, especially when access to the patient is limited, e.g. during neuro- or craniofacial surgery or surgical interventions performed with the patient in the prone position. In the presented case of a patient with gastroschisis, a prolonged period of parenteral nutrition could be expected, and therefore central venous access to an internal jugular or a subclavian vein seemed preferable.

After **gastroschisis** repair, feeding tolerance develops only very slowly, and central venous access for parenteral nutrition is always required. In contrast to omphalocoele, gastroschisis is usually not associated with other congenital malformations. Nevertheless, it has been the author's practice to request echocardiography in all neonates presenting for major surgery. Should haemodynamic instability occur, it is reassuring to know that there are no structural cardiac anomalies. Gastroschisis repair increases the intra-abdominal pressure, potentially leading to an abdominal compartment syndrome. Based on a few published cases, it is generally believed that the intra-abdominal pressure should be measured, e.g. by measuring gastric or bladder pressure, and that abdominal closure should be delayed if this pressure is above 20 mmHg (Yaster *et al.* 1988).

Summary and Recommendations

When central venous access is obtained through puncture of internal jugular, subclavian or brachiocephalic veins, there is always a risk of causing a pneumothorax. Timely recognition and treatment are important to avoid potential long-term consequences.

For short-term use, a femoral approach for central venous access is a good option, because it minimizes puncture-related complications.

References

Breschan, C., Platzer, M., Jost, R., *et al.* (2007). Comparison of catheter-related infection and tip colonization between internal jugular and subclavian central venous catheters in surgical neonates. *Anesthesiology*, 107, 946–953.

Bruschettini, M., Romantsik, O., Ramenghi, L.A., *et al.* (2016). Needle aspiration versus intercostal tube drainage for pneumothorax in the newborn. *Cochrane Database Syst Rev*, (1), CD011724.

Camkiran, F.A., Zeyneloglu, P., Ozkan, M., *et al.* (2016). A randomized controlled comparison of the internal jugular vein and the subclavian vein as access sites for central venous catheterization in pediatric cardiac surgery. *Pediatr Crit Care Med*, 17, e413–e419.

Cattarossi, L., Copetti, R., Brusa, G., *et al.* (2016). Lung ultrasound diagnostic accuracy in neonatal pneumothorax. *Can Respir J*, 2016, 6515069. http://dx.doi.org/10.1155/2016/6515069 (accessed 29 November 2017).

Kuhns, L.R., Bednarek, F.J., Wyman, M.L., *et al.* (1975). Diagnosis of pneumothorax or pneumomediastinum in the neonate by transillumination. *Pediatrics*, 56, 355–360.

Liu, J., Chi, J.H., Ren, X.L., *et al.* (2017). Lung ultrasonography to diagnose pneumothorax of the newborn. *Am J Emerg Med*, 35, 1298–1302.

Ruesch, S., Walder, B., & Tramèr, M.R. (2002). Complications of central venous catheters: internal jugular versus subclavian access: a systematic review. *Crit Care Med*, 30, 454–460.

Yaster, M., Buck, J.R., Dudgeon, D.L., *et al.* (1988). Hemodynamic effects of primary closure of omphalocele/gastroschisis in human newborns. *Anesthesiology*, 69, 84–88.

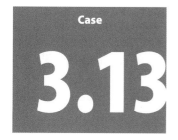

Post-Obstructive Pulmonary Oedema

Case

A 13-year-old girl, weighing 50 kg, was scheduled for repair of a residual defect after cleft palate repair in early infancy. After inhalational induction, venous access was obtained, she was intubated with a cuffed oral RAE tube size 7.0, and anaesthesia was then maintained with isoflurane, fentanyl and repeated doses of atracurium.

At the completion of surgery, the surgeon applied a dressing with a gauze dipped in a doughy synthetic fluid. Ten minutes later, at full recovery from neuromuscular blockade, isoflurane was turned off. She rapidly opened her eyes and tried to pull out the endotracheal tube (ETT). After extubation, she became very agitated and her venous access accidentally got lost. Severe inspiratory airway obstruction was now apparent, with massive stridor and only minimal air entry to the lungs. These symptoms persisted for several minutes despite the positive airway pressure and 100% oxygen via face mask and attempts to calm her.

After re-establishing venous access, thiopental and succinylcholine were injected and orotracheal intubation was attempted but initially unsuccessful. Despite repeated suctioning, a huge foamy mushroom of slightly pinkish secretions emerged from her mouth. Intubation was finally successful and the patient was transferred to the intensive care unit. Clinically and radiologically, signs of massive pulmonary oedema were evident. Initial ventilator settings were remarkable, with an FiO_2 of 80% and a PEEP of 10 cmH$_2$O. Both parameters could be gradually weaned, and the need for repeated suctioning diminished over the next few hours. The next morning, she was ready for extubation.

Surprisingly, her stridor persisted, until, on postoperative day 5, she coughed out a cast of the laryngeal inlet made from the plastic material that had been used for the dressing.

Discussion

This case illustrates the typical clinical consequences of **post-obstructive pulmonary oedema**, also called negative-pressure pulmonary oedema or pulmonary oedema ex vacuo. Its pathophysiology is not completely understood (Bhattacharya *et al.* 2016, Yemen 2000). Probably, massive negative intra-alveolar pressure during inspiration against resistance causes fluid shift from the capillaries into the interstitial space and later into the alveolar space (Fremont *et al.* 2007). This hydrostatic phenomenon leads to alveolar fluid accumulation with a low protein content (Devys *et al.* 2000b). The fluid may wash out and dilute surfactant, leading to alveolar collapse and impaired oxygenation. This phenomenon typically occurs in adolescents or young adults who are able to generate massive inspiratory efforts. Many cases occur after ENT or maxillofacial surgery, interventions typically

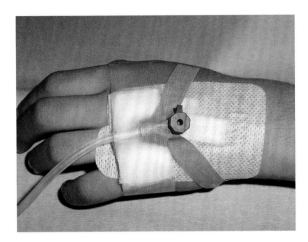

Figure 3.13 Venous access has to be secured before emergence from anaesthesia. The figure illustrates the currently used standard method at the Children's Hospital in Lucerne.

associated with postoperative airway obstruction and laryngospasm. Even biting on the artificial airway can cause negative-pressure pulmonary oedema (Devys *et al.* 2000a).

Treatment focuses on relieving the upper airway obstruction and maintaining oxygenation. Re-intubation is typically required, and CPAP or PEEP is needed to recruit the lungs and diminish intrapulmonary shunting. As there is no absolute fluid overload, the value of diuretics in this condition is questionable, although they are often used (Austin *et al.* 2016, Sharma & Singh 2008). Improvement requires re-establishment of the alveolar barrier including surfactant, which usually takes some hours. Radiological improvement typically lags behind clinical improvement. Therefore, when the diagnosis is clear, follow-up x-rays are not helpful to determine when the patient can be extubated.

Prevention of post-obstructive pulmonary oedema requires prevention of any type of airway obstruction, especially in spontaneously breathing children. If airway obstruction occurs, e.g. laryngospasm or an occluded airway by a patient biting on the ETT, rapid treatment is mandatory and any delay may be dangerous.

An additional educational aspect of the presented case involves the **loss of intravenous access** right at the beginning just as the problem developed. The venous cannula was not yet fixed using tape and the application of a splint, as defined by the standard operating procedures in the author's institution (Fig. 3.13). Venous access has to be secured before a patient emerges from anaesthesia.

Initially, the prolonged stay in the intensive care unit was interpreted as the consequence of an anaesthesia-related complication. Undoubtedly, it was in fact due to the foreign material that dropped down into the larynx, causing protracted laryngospasm and persistent stridor. After every intraoral procedure, extreme care must be taken to ensure that no foreign bodies go unrecognised.

Summary and Recommendations

The presented case of post-obstructive pulmonary oedema emphasizes the role of prevention and rapid treatment of upper airway obstruction.

Any venous access has to be secured so that it cannot get lost in case of a stormy emergence. A more timely intervention might have prevented the development of massive pulmonary oedema.

It is remarkable that the true cause of post-obstructive pulmonary oedema, i.e. surgical material at the laryngeal inlet, only became apparent after several days. Up to this point, the parents were convinced that the complication was purely anaesthesia-related. When explaining unexpected and unexplained adverse events to parents, careful wording is advisable.

References

Austin, A.L., Kon, A., & Matteucci, M.J. (2016). Respiratory failure in a child due to type 2 postobstructive pulmonary edema. *Pediatr Emerg Care*, 32, 23–24.

Bhattacharya, M., Kallet, R.H., Ware, L.B., *et al.* (2016). Negative-pressure pulmonary edema. *Chest*, 150, 927–933.

Devys, J.M., Balleau, C., Jayr, C., *et al.* (2000a). Biting the laryngeal mask: an unusual cause of negative pressure pulmonary edema. *Can J Anaesth*, 47, 176–178.

Devys, J.M., Cadi, P., & Nivoche, Y. (2000b). Protein concentration in pulmonary oedema fluid for negative pressure pulmonary oedema in children. *Paediatr Anaesth*, 10, 557–558.

Fremont, R.D., Kallet, R.H., Matthay, M.A., *et al.* (2007). Postobstructive pulmonary edema: a case for hydrostatic mechanisms. *Chest*, 131, 1742–1746.

Sharma, P. & Singh, B. (2008). Fluid restriction in the management of postobstructive pulmonary edema: wise or otherwise? *J Clin Anesth*, 20, 155–156.

Yemen, T.A. (2000). How much do we really know about postobstructive pulmonary oedema? *Paediatr Anaesth*, 10, 459–461.

Pulmonary Aspiration

Case

An 11-year-old girl, weighing 30 kg, with a history of intermittent abdominal pain and obstipation, was scheduled for rectal examination and stool evacuation. Her past medical history was remarkable for congenital diaphragmatic hernia with a prolonged stay in the neonatal intensive care unit. Currently, she experienced no limitations during normal daily life, but walking uphill rapidly caused dyspnoea. She reported no pain, no nausea and the abdomen did not appear to be distended. After oral premedication with midazolam and local application of EMLA cream an intravenous induction was planned. However, the girl insisted that she would not tolerate venous cannulation.

Therefore, anaesthesia was induced by mask with 70% nitrous oxide and 8% sevoflurane. Sixty seconds later breathing stopped and a small amount of clear fluid briefly appeared in the corner of her mouth. Breathing efforts restarted and massive laryngospasm developed with paradoxical excursions of the thorax. Despite an open airway, 100% oxygen and high airway pressures, oxygen saturation rapidly fell below 90%. Mask ventilation was ineffective. After venous cannulation and the administration of rocuronium 1 mg/kg, the trachea was intubated uneventfully using a size 6.0 cuffed endotracheal tube (ETT). However, ventilation and oxygenation proved to be difficult, requiring a peak pressure of 30 cmH$_2$O and a PEEP of 10 cmH$_2$O; despite an FiO$_2$ of 100%, oxygen saturation remained below 90%. Fibreoptic inspection of the bronchial tree showed no particular material or coloured secretions.

After the insertion of an arterial line and a central venous catheter, the patient was transferred to the paediatric intensive care unit (PICU). The chest x-ray showed bilateral infiltrations (Fig. 3.14), which resolved only in part over the next 72 hours. However, radiologically a recurrent diaphragmatic hernia was suspected. Three days later, while she was still dependent on mechanical ventilatory support with an FiO$_2$ of 40%, laparotomy was performed and part of the colon was found to be trapped in a gap of the diaphragm.

Discussion

In this case, **aspiration** of clear acid gastric content during mask induction was the most likely cause of laryngospasm and respiratory decompensation. Only clear fluid was seen at the corner of the mouth, and early bronchoscopy showed no signs of other aspirated material, especially no traces of coloured or particulate material. This aspiration event was clearly not benign; it caused severe respiratory failure necessitating

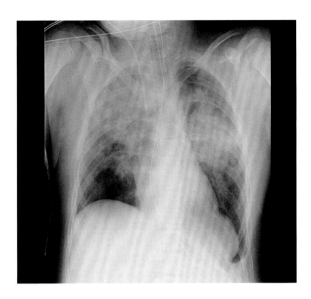

Figure 3.14 Chest x-ray taken 2 hours after the event showed bilateral pulmonary infiltrations. In addition, the left diaphragm had a striking configuration. At surgery, part of the colon was found to be trapped in a gap of the repaired diaphragm.

mechanical ventilation for several days with an FiO_2 of 60–80% and high PEEP settings. One could speculate that some degree of residual lung hypoplasia and pulmonary hypertension secondary to congenital diaphragmatic hernia could have aggravated the clinical course.

Initially, post-obstructive pulmonary oedema (cf. Case 3.13) was considered to be a possible **differential diagnosis**. The preceding impressive laryngospasm with forceful but unsuccessful inspiratory efforts could lead to post-obstructive pulmonary oedema with similar chest x-ray findings and severely impaired gas exchange, as seen in the presented patient. However, the prolonged course over several days and complete absence of foamy sputum argue against this diagnosis.

Would it have been possible to anticipate the **risk of pulmonary aspiration** in this patient? A history of intermittent abdominal pain and constipation is suspicious. On the other hand, the abdomen was not distended, there were no distended loops of bowel on abdominal x-ray (not shown) and, at the time of induction, no pain or nausea was present. Therefore, the anaesthetist's decision to proceed with inhalational induction when the girl expressed her fears seems quite defensible.

Pulmonary aspiration is a real threat in paediatric anaesthesia (Borland *et al.* 1998, Walker 2013, Warner *et al.* 1999). In children, fatal cases are very rare, but, as illustrated by the presented case, morbidity can be significant (Lussmann & Gerber 1997). Therefore, rapid sequence induction should not be trivialized in children. Every effort should be made to avoid aspiration, and only apnoea should not be part of the paediatric protocol (Engelhardt 2015, Jöhr 2007). In a classical series, the incidence of aspiration has been reported to be 1:2632 in elective patients and 10 times higher in emergency cases (Warner *et al.* 1999). In a medical system, where almost all patients were managed by experienced consultant paediatric anaesthetists, a lower incidence of 1:5000 was reported (Walker 2013). However, in a recent pan-European study, the incidence was 1:1000 (Habre *et al.* 2017), similar to a more historical series two decades ago (Borland *et al.* 1998).

In case of a suspected aspiration event the following steps should be followed:

- First, identification of the aspirated material to assess the risk of damage, and, in intubated children, bronchoscopy to rule out aspiration of particulate material.
- Second, minimizing damage by suctioning both mouth and airway, and, if needed, securing the airway with an ETT.
- Third, maintaining adequate oxygenation by oxygen administration, positive airway pressure and recruitment manoeuvres.

Prophylactic intubation and ventilation does not alter the course of the disease, and endotracheal intubation should be performed only when indicated by impaired gas exchange or persistent risk of aspiration. Measures which are potentially harmful and therefore to be avoided include bronchial lavage, instillation of alkalinizing fluids and repeated forceful suctioning. The administration of corticosteroids is of no proven use. Antibiotics are indicated if contaminated material has been aspirated. In many cases, the precise nature of the aspirated material remains unknown; it is a pragmatic approach to administer antibiotics in children with persistent clinical or radiological signs of aspiration and to de-escalate rapidly following resolution. In contrast to adults, prognosis in children is usually favourable. When no signs or symptoms appear within 1–2 hours after an aspiration event, a benign course is very likely (Walker 2013, Warner *et al.* 1999).

Summary and Recommendations

This case of gastric acid aspiration leading to severe impairment of pulmonary gas exchange with prolonged stay in the intensive care unit illustrates that pulmonary aspiration is a persistent threat, even if mortality in this usually otherwise healthy population rarely occurs.

Every effort should be made to avoid such events in children by using a modified rapid sequence induction, which includes all necessary precautions to avoid regurgitation, but recommends gentle mask ventilation before endotracheal intubation in order to avoid hypoxaemia.

This case also illustrates that even after careful preoperative evaluation of risk factors by an experienced team, severe complications can occur.

References

Borland, L.M., Sereika, S.M., Woelfel, S.K., *et al.* (1998). Pulmonary aspiration in pediatric patients during general anesthesia: incidence and outcome. *J Clin Anesth*, 10, 95–102.

Engelhardt, T. (2015). Rapid sequence induction has no use in pediatric anesthesia. *Paediatr Anaesth*, 25, 5–8.

Habre, W., Disma, N., Virag, K., *et al.* (2017). Incidence of severe critical events in paediatric anaesthesia (APRICOT): a prospective multicentre observational study in 261 hospitals in Europe. *Lancet Respir Med*, 5, 412–425.

Jöhr, M. (2007). Anaesthesia for the child with a full stomach. *Curr Opin Anaesthesiol*, 20, 201–203.

Lussmann, R.F. & Gerber, H.R. (1997). Severe aspiration pneumonia with the laryngeal mask [in German]. *Anasthesiol Intensivmed Notfallmed Schmerzther*, 32, 194–196.

Walker, R.W. (2013). Pulmonary aspiration in pediatric anesthetic practice in the UK: a prospective survey of specialist pediatric centers over a one-year period. *Paediatr Anaesth*, 23, 702–711.

Warner, M.A., Warner, M.E., Warner, D.O., *et al.* (1999). Perioperative pulmonary aspiration in infants and children. *Anesthesiology*, 90, 66–71.

Bronchial Foreign Body

Case

A long time ago, a 2-day-old term female neonate with cleft palate was scheduled as an additional case for monitored anaesthesia care for a cleft palate impression procedure in the late afternoon (Fig. 3.15a). At the end of a busy list, everybody felt relieved when it was announced that the girl had been taken directly to the maxillofacial department by mistake. There, the cleft palate impression had been taken uneventfully.

Two days later, the now 4-day-old neonate was transferred from the regular ward to the neonatal intensive care unit because of severe respiratory distress. She presented with a respiratory rate of over 80 breaths per minute and an additional oxygen requirement. The chest x-ray revealed a right-sided tension pneumothorax, which was relieved by needle aspiration through a 24G plastic cannula. The clinical condition improved, but follow-up x-ray still showed infiltrations in the right lower lobe. Understandably, as these events occurred in the middle of the night, the possible association between the cleft palate impression procedure and tension pneumothorax was not immediately obvious to the staff on call.

The following day, another chest x-ray was obtained, and this confirmed re-expansion of the right lung but persistence of right lower lobe infiltrations. The girl was transferred to the operating theatre for bronchoscopy under general anaesthesia. The procedure was started with flexible bronchoscopy through a laryngeal mask airway (LMA) size 1; this was followed by extraction of a large foreign body with a length of almost 3 cm from the right main-stem bronchus through a rigid bronchoscope (Fig. 3.15b). The patient made a rapid recovery and her further hospital course was uneventful.

Retrospectively, it was reported that during the impression procedure there had been a short episode of severe coughing, which subsided rapidly.

Discussion

This case illustrates that there is always a risk that **foreign material** in the oral cavity can be aspirated. The slightest suspicion of an aspiration event should trigger early bronchoscopy. In cases of suspected foreign body aspiration, it is a rational approach to begin with fibreoptic bronchoscopy through an LMA or by using the Frei endoscopy mask (Frei *et al.* 1995). In addition to inspection of the bronchial tree, the latter device provides an excellent view of the piriform sinus and the supraglottic region. When spontaneous breathing is maintained, it also allows functional evaluation to rule out vocal cord paralysis, laryngomalacia or tracheomalacia. However, before passing the vocal cords, local anaesthesia or neuromuscular blockade is recommended. Fibreoptic inspection is less invasive than

(a)

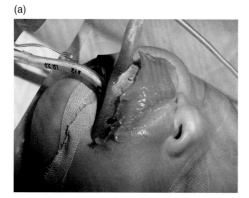

(b)

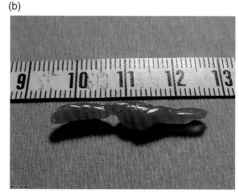

Figure 3.15a The cleft palate impression procedure in an intubated neonate.

Figure 3.15b Material extracted from the right main-stem bronchus two days after a cleft palate impression procedure in the awake neonate.

rigid bronchoscopy and will cause less airway irritation. Rigid bronchoscopy is only performed when a foreign body has been identified.

Typically, children with **foreign body aspiration** are between 1 and 4 years of age. In this age group, food particles, e.g. nuts, seeds or parts of carrots, are often encountered. But all age groups and all types of non-food particles can be involved as well. In the very young child, another person is usually involved: siblings trying to feed a neonate, or, as in this case, medical staff. In symptomatic patients, and in very young children, **timely bronchoscopy** and extraction on the urgent list are recommended, because dislodgement can lead to fatal complete airway obstruction.

The risk of severe complications following foreign body aspiration should not be under-estimated. In a recent large series, a mortality rate of 2.5% was reported (Johnson *et al.* 2017). In older children, who are asymptomatic at rest, especially when the suspicious event occurred several days ago, it seems acceptable to schedule the case on the next day on a regular list.

For some but not all maxillofacial surgeons, the occlusion of the cleft by a **plate** is part of the treatment concept for cleft lip and palate repair. The plate is meant to improve oral feeding, protect the middle ear from contamination, and prevent the tongue from falling back. Theoretically, this could also facilitate mandibular growth. However, there is no consensus about the clinical efficacy or the importance of this treatment step, and the large majority of infants with cleft lip and palate can be fed without such a device.

To produce the plate, a **cleft palate impression** procedure is required. In neonates, this is not without risks (Chate 1994). In a historical audit involving 193 consultants, 89 reported cyanotic spells, 89 relevant difficulties and 4 cases of asphyxia; fortunately, no death was reported (Chate 1995). In a more recent series, the administration of oxygen and the presence of an anaesthetist was recommended (Nur *et al.* 2016). It has repeatedly been emphasized that extreme care is needed when the procedure is performed in neonates (Dubey *et al.* 2013). An informal audit among paediatric anaesthetists in the German-speaking part of Europe showed that a majority was unaware of the potential procedure-related problems, which may indicate that many neonates are treated in physicians' or dentists' offices. In some institutions, neonatologists monitor these patients during the procedure. A few colleagues recommended general endotracheal anaesthesia. Triggered by the presented case, the author began to exclusively use general endotracheal anaesthesia. It should be emphasized that only a thorough inspection of the pharyngeal cavity down to the larynx prior to extubation protects against aspiration of lost impression material.

Summary and Recommendations

This case illustrates that foreign body aspiration is a real threat in neonates and young children, and requires timely investigation.

Rigid bronchoscopy under general anaesthesia is the recommended technique for foreign body extraction; but initially, especially if there is the slightest doubt about the diagnosis, fibreoptic bronchoscopy may be preferable because it causes less irritation to the airway and provides a better view.

This story also demonstrates that potentially risky manoeuvres, such as instilling a semiliquid substance into the mouth of a neonate, are often performed injudiciously, because it has always been done this way and because the individual physician has never encountered severe complications of these rarely performed procedures.

References

Chate, R.A. (1994). Respiratory arrest during an orthodontic impression of a cleft palate, in a baby with Brachmann-de Lange syndrome. *J R Coll Surg Edinb*, 39, 121–123.

Chate, R.A. (1995). A report on the hazards encountered when taking neonatal cleft palate impressions (1983–1992). *Br J Orthod*, 22, 299–307.

Dubey, A., Mujoo, S., Khandelwal, V., *et al.* (2013). Simplified design and precautionary measures in fabrication of a feeding obturator for a newborn with cleft lip and palate. *BMJ Case Rep*, 2013. pii: bcr2013010465. doi: 10.1136/bcr-2013-010465.

Frei, F.J., aWengen, D.F., Rutishauser, M., *et al.* (1995). The airway endoscopy mask: useful device for fibreoptic evaluation and intubation of the paediatric airway. *Paediatr Anaesth*, 5, 319–324.

Johnson, K., Linnaus, M., & Notrica, D. (2017). Airway foreign bodies in pediatric patients: anatomic location of foreign body affects complications and outcomes. *Pediatr Surg Int*, 33, 59–64.

Nur, R.B., Cakan, D.G., & Noyan, A. (2016). Evaluation of oxygen saturation and heart rate during intraoral impression taking in infants with cleft lip and palate. *J Craniofac Surg*, 27, e118–e121.

Pharyngeal Foreign Body

Case

A 9-year-old girl was scheduled for revision surgery after cleft lip and palate repair. Anaesthesia was induced by mask with sevoflurane and nitrous oxide; after mivacurium 0.2 mg/kg followed by an infusion, the trachea was intubated with a 6.5 cuffed RAE tube. After endotracheal intubation sevoflurane was replaced by desflurane and fentanyl was given for analgesia. The surgeon infiltrated the field with bupivacaine 0.25% with adrenaline to reduce bleeding; additionally clonidine 2 μg/kg was administered to increase the likelihood of a quiet recovery.

At the end of surgery, desflurane was turned off and the pharynx was suctioned. The girl opened her eyes, showed adequate tidal volumes and was extubated. After a few undisturbed breaths, signs of upper airway obstruction became apparent. The girl became severely dyspnoeic. Repeat suctioning of the pharynx and administration of 100% oxygen by face mask applying positive airway pressure did not improve the situation. Direct laryngoscopy was attempted in the now struggling child, but allowed no clear view of the larynx because everything was red and had a blood-tinged appearance. Suddenly, she was gagging and expelled a red piece of 'tissue', which proved to be a swab (Fig. 3.16). This was followed by unobstructed breathing, and the patient calmed down and became cooperative.

Discussion

This case of a lost swab in the pharynx, which almost led to suffocation, emphasizes the importance of carefully inspecting the pharynx after every intraoral intervention. In case of airway obstruction following an intraoral intervention, **iatrogenic pharyngeal foreign bodies** should always be part of the differential diagnosis. The author remembers several similar events during his professional career. In oral surgery, meticulous care is needed to avoid the loss of parts of medical devices or swabs in the oral cavity. Swabs or gauzes coming into contact with the surgical field rapidly become blood-tinged and reddish and thus, at a first glance, difficult to distinguish from the mucosa. It is part of the safety concept that all swabs left intraorally are marked with a suture, which is led out of the mouth. However, in reality, surgical colleagues often ignore this because they feel disturbed by the suture passing through the operative field.

Pharyngeal foreign bodies can make **ventilation by mask difficult or impossible**. Therefore, laryngoscopy to search for a foreign body should be part of every algorithm dealing with the **unexpected difficult airway** in children (Weiss & Engelhardt 2010). Vivid imagination is needed to list all possible objects that can be found in the mouth of a child. During laryngoscopy for the routine induction of a child the author has encountered, quite

(a)

(b)

(c)

(d)

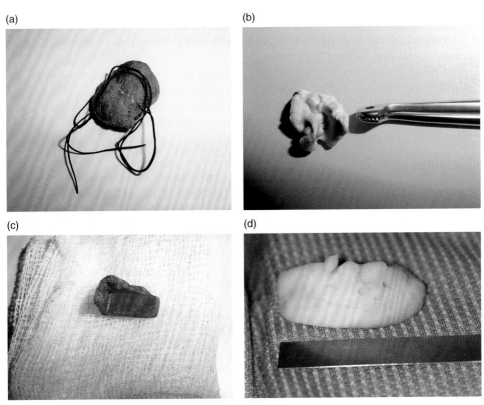

Figure 3.16 Various pharyngeal foreign bodies can be encountered in patients with symptoms of upper airway obstruction: **(a)** surgical swab (responsible in the case presented here), **(b)** chewing gum found at laryngoscopy, **(c)** a piece of plastic, **(d)** a piece of an apple leading to almost complete airway obstruction.

unexpectedly, a piece of chewing gum lying between the vocal cords (Fig. 3.16). In another case, a toddler was deeply sedated for more than an hour during a prolonged procedure under regional anaesthesia, when he suddenly began to snore, then to gag until he finally coughed out a large piece of plastic probably belonging to a toy. Food particles (e.g. part of an apple) can also be encountered and, with the exception of the signs of infection, clinically mimic signs and symptoms of acute epiglottitis. Such patients can present with signs of inspiratory airway obstruction, drooling, disturbed voice (so-called 'hot potato voice') and an extended and open mouth. Parts of airway devices can become disconnected as well (Soong *et al.* 2010). The threat of suffocation is always present in young children (Lifschultz & Donoghue 1996).

In patients with unclear airway obstruction, it is the author's practice to induce anaesthesia by mask with sevoflurane in 100% oxygen while maintaining spontaneous ventilation as long as possible and then performing laryngoscopy to make sure that the laryngeal entrance can be identified. Surprisingly, when applying a positive airway pressure of 5–10 cm H_2O, in several dozens of cases, airway obstruction has never been a problem. Obviously, distending the upper airway with positive pressure in a quiet, spontaneously breathing child is always helpful. In contrast, without CPAP, and especially in an agitated child, the epiglottis or the foreign body can be sucked into the laryngeal entrance and can cause complete airway obstruction.

Summary and Recommendations

A pharyngeal foreign body should always be part of the differential diagnosis in a child presenting with upper airway obstruction.

Following oral surgery, meticulous care is needed to remove all foreign materials; the oral cavity must be thoroughly suctioned and carefully inspected.

The presented case also illustrates that physicians sometimes do not follow recommended safety precautions, even though potential complications could be fatal.

References

Lifschultz, B.D. & Donoghue, E.R. (1996). Deaths due to foreign body aspiration in children: the continuing hazard of toy balloons. *J Forensic Sci*, 41, 247–251.

Soong, W.J., Lee, Y.S., Soong, Y.H., *et al.* (2010). Tracheal foreign body after laser supraglottoplasty: a hidden but risky complication of an aluminum foil tape-wrapped endotracheal tube. *Int J Pediatr Otorhinolaryngol*, 74, 1432–1434.

Weiss, M. & Engelhardt, T. (2010). Proposal for the management of the unexpected difficult pediatric airway. *Paediatr Anaesth*, 20, 454–464.

Oesophageal Foreign Body

Case

Many decades ago, in a small district hospital, a child was born at 36 weeks of gestation by urgent caesarean section because of placental abruption. The 2000 g neonate was pale and flaccid, and no pulse was felt at the base of the umbilical cord. The mother was under general anaesthesia and the anaesthetist handed her over to the nurse to be able to attend to the neonate. After some hectic minutes and several attempts at orotracheal intubation, resuscitation of the neonate was ultimately successful.

For the transfer to the neonatal intensive care unit (NICU) in Lucerne, a senior staff neonatologist was called and arrived with an ambulance. He chose to change the endo-tracheal tube (ETT) from its orotracheal to a nasotracheal position prior to transport. On arrival in the NICU, the patient was already on minimal respiratory support. A chest x-ray showed a gastric tube in place and bilateral diminished lung aeration. The patient could be extubated within 24 hours, and was transferred back to the birth clinic on day 4 of life.

Six weeks later, the physician in charge of the baby again requested transfer of the patient because of feeding difficulties and suspected brain damage. The baby now weighed 2800 g. Brain ultrasound examination and polysomnography were normal. An upper gastrointestinal contrast study was ordered because of suspected gastro-oesophageal reflux. A large oesophageal foreign body had already been identified on a plain-view radiograph (Fig. 3.17). The infant was taken to theatre and anaesthetized, and a size 3.0 Portex ETT without connector was extracted. The patient made a full and uneventful recovery and rapidly gained weight. He was seen again for inguinal hernia repair at the age of 5 months. Part of this story has previously been reported (Jöhr & Schubiger 1995).

Discussion

This case of **a lost ETT** illustrates that even a large foreign body can remain undetected in the oesophagus for weeks or even months, if no one thinks of it. It also shows that a partially awake individual can reflexively swallow foreign bodies when they have arrived in the pharynx; this has been described for ETTs (Block *et al.* 1999, Dickson & Fraser 1967, Gronczewski 2005, Wu *et al.* 1997), dentures (Kent *et al.* 2016), Guedel airways and even laryngeal mask airways (LMAs). The author once induced a girl weighing 31 kg by mask and inserted a classic type LMA size 3 by the rotational technique, but, because anaesthesia was too superficial, the girl swallowed forcefully and the LMA disappeared behind the tongue. At the very last moment it could be retrieved with a Kocher's forceps. Surprisingly, there are not only numerous case reports of swallowed ETTs, but aspiration is also possible, especially when an ETT that is much too small is chosen (Durall *et al.* 2003, Wong *et al.* 2003).

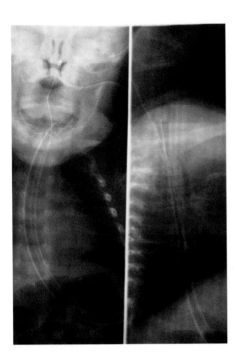

Figure 3.17 Six weeks after neonatal resuscitation, a large foreign body, compatible with an ETT, was seen during fluoroscopy while evaluating the patient for gastro-oesophageal reflux (left panel, anteroposterior view; right panel, lateral view).

Oesophageal foreign bodies can be a major threat to the patient. Large objects can completely impede feeding or create an airway obstruction (Kim *et al.* 2008). **Button batteries** are particularly dangerous because with mucosal contact the electric circuit is closed and the current causes deep mucosal damage that can lead to oesophageal perforation (Leinwand *et al.* 2016). Emergency endoscopy and immediate removal is mandatory. According to current guidelines, it is dangerous to wait until the usual fasting period has elapsed. After several days, the removal of button batteries becomes more difficult because of massive tissue reaction, even if there is no perforation. The author remembers a case in which the surgeon had to proceed to cervical oesophagotomy for removal. A special challenge is the removal of sharp objects, such as open safety pins or metallic stars.

In case of **unobserved ingestion** of foreign bodies, this possibility is often not considered. The author remembers a 2 6/12-year-old girl with a coin lodged behind the cricoid at the entrance of the oesophagus, who was treated with antibiotics for several weeks for presumed bronchitis, until she was finally transferred to the children's hospital because of weight loss and fever.

We can all be misled by **having the wrong focus**. Therefore, in critical situations, teamwork becomes even more important because it can give rise to divergent ideas and opinions. While critically reviewing this case, it is obvious that early diagnosis would have been possible. On the initial chest x-ray the endotracheal tube lying in the oesophagus was clearly visible. However, all staff members expected to see a nasogastric tube, so even the radiologist described a nasogastric tube. The description of 'snoring respiration' and 'appearance of gagging' described in the nursing protocol was also ignored. It is of the utmost importance that all clinical findings are seen and interpreted with a **completely open mind**. At least initially, a wide differential diagnosis, including even very rare alternatives, should be considered. As on a radar screen, where not every point is necessarily an airplane, other objects must be considered. As a rule, we only recognize objects and diagnose disorders we have known or seen before.

Summary and Recommendations

This case shows that even obvious findings, like the clearly visible ETT on the initial chest x-ray in the presented patient, are sometimes not recognized when they are not expected. This emphasizes the importance of a wide differential diagnosis and a completely open mind.

Accidental swallowing of even large foreign bodies can occur, especially in partially conscious patients.

References

Block, E.F., Cheatham, M.L., Parrish, G.A., et al. (1999). Ingested endotracheal tube in an adult following intubation attempt for head injury. *Am Surg*, 65, 1134–1136.

Dickson, J.A. & Fraser, G.C. (1967). 'Swallowed' endotracheal tube: a new neonatal emergency. *Br Med J*, 2, (5555), 811–812.

Durall, A., Bertha, R.J., & Slusher, T. (2003). An unusual complication of endotracheal intubation. *Respir Care*, 48, 522–523.

Gronczewski, C.A. (2005). The lost endotracheal tube: an unreported complication of prehospital intubation. *Pediatr Emerg Care*, 21, 318–321.

Jöhr, M. & Schubiger, G. (1995). The lost tracheal tube: a rare complication of failed intubation. *Paediatr Anaesth*, 5, 397–398.

Kent, S.J., Mackie, J., & Macfarlane, T.V. (2016). Designing for safety: implications of a fifteen year review of swallowed and aspirated dentures. *J Oral Maxillofac Res*, 7, e3.

Kim, N., Atkinson, N., & Manicone, P. (2008). Esophageal foreign body: a case of a neonate with stridor. *Pediatr Emerg Care*, 24, 849–851.

Leinwand, K., Brumbaugh, D.E., & Kramer, R.E. (2016). Button battery ingestion in children: a paradigm for management of severe pediatric foreign body ingestions. *Gastrointest Endosc Clin N Am*, 26, 99–118.

Wong, S.Y., Tseng, C.H., Wong, K.M., et al. (2003). Aspiration of a dislodged endotracheal tube: a rare cause of acute total airway obstruction. *Chang Gung Med J*, 26, 515–519.

Wu, C.T., Li, C.Y., Wong, C.S., et al. (1997). The lost endotracheal tube: a rare complication of accidental esophageal intubation. *Acta Anaesthesiol Sin*, 35, 55–58.

Case 3.18

Unanticipated Tracheal Stenosis

Case

A long time ago, an almost 3-year-old boy was scheduled for tonsillectomy because of suspected obstructive sleep apnoea. He was induced intravenously with thiopental, alfentanil and atracurium. Face-mask ventilation was easily achieved. The anaesthesia resident tried to intubate with a size 5.0 uncuffed preformed endotracheal tube (ETT) but failed; he reported that he had seen the glottis but that the ETT would not pass. The head nurse took over and was also unsuccessful. Therefore, smaller ETTs were tried, but even the alerted attending anaesthetist was unsuccessful in inserting a size 3.5 ETT despite good visibility of the glottis. When the paediatric anaesthetist and ENT surgeon arrived, the diagnosis of a critical airway stenosis now aggravated by swelling was made. Given the increasingly difficult mask ventilation and the history of multiple trials of unsuccessful intubation, tracheotomy was felt to be indicated.

An 8F Cook airway-exchange catheter could be passed through the narrowing of the trachea and connected via extension tubing to a manual jet ventilator (Manujet). A few puffs restored oxygenation and the child was now ventilated manually with this device, with visible chest movements. The inhalational anaesthetic was replaced by a propofol infusion. After draping the surgical field, which impeded observation of the chest, bradycardia suddenly developed, accompanied by a weak radial pulse. Because lung overdistension was suspected, jet ventilation was interrupted, the patient was disconnected and manual compression of the thorax resulted in a slow escape of gas with a wheezing noise. Jet ventilation was then resumed with much shorter puffs at a lower frequency; nevertheless, a second episode occurred, which was treated in an identical way. Only when the surgeon had incised the trachea, allowing air to escape, could manual jet ventilation be resumed in an ordinary way.

The boy later underwent laryngeal laser surgery and insertion of a T-tube as a stent because of a congenital subglottic stenosis.

Discussion

This case of an unexpected subglottic **laryngeal stenosis** illustrates that multiple attempts of intubation can cause harm and induce swelling. In such situations, it is important to find out why the tube cannot be advanced into the trachea, e.g. by inserting a laryngeal mask airway (LMA) and fibreoptic inspection.

Manual jet ventilation is a rescue technique in case of failed intubation; however, in emergency situations, even in adults, failure and complication rates are quite high (Duggan *et al.* 2016), especially when percutaneous puncture of the airway is used. Percutaneous puncture of the trachea is not recommended in children (Weiss & Engelhardt 2010), but translaryngeal insertion of a catheter may be an option (cf. Case 3.8). With jet ventilation a sufficient amount of oxygen can be instilled into the lungs with each puff even through a very thin catheter, e.g. a 20G venous cannula. This allows the patient to be kept alive for a prolonged period provided that the remaining space around the catheter is wide enough to allow sufficient passive exhalation; otherwise overdistension of the lungs can lead to barotrauma and, as in the presented case, impede pulmonary blood flow resulting in cardiovascular collapse. Extreme care has to be taken not to insert the catheter too deeply, because, when it slips into a wedge position, a pneumothorax will almost inevitably occur. For the same reason, insufflation of oxygen through the biopsy channel of a flexible bronchoscope is strongly discouraged in young children: the risk that the relatively large-sized bronchoscope will completely impede exhalation at some point in the procedure is just too high (Chan & Gamble 2016). It is likely that **Ventrain**, a system which also supports expiration (Willemsen *et al.* 2014), will replace conventional manual jet ventilation devices in the near future. Ventrain really allows ventilation 'through a straw' independent of sufficient space for passive exhalation (Hamaekers *et al.* 2015).

Tonsillectomy was indicated because of a history of noisy breathing and night-time snoring. About 8–15% of all children snore, but only 1–4% have **obstructive sleep apnoea** (Gursanscky *et al.* 2017). Large tonsils are a sensitive but non-specific finding (Certal *et al.* 2012). An increasing number of parents record videos with their smartphones documenting observed apnoea when the child unsuccessfully tries to breathe. Additional symptoms are a disturbed and restless sleep combined with daytime sleepiness. If there is any doubt about the diagnosis, polysomnography is the gold standard to confirm or exclude obstructive sleep apnoea (Marcus *et al.* 2012). In reality, in many children the diagnosis is based solely

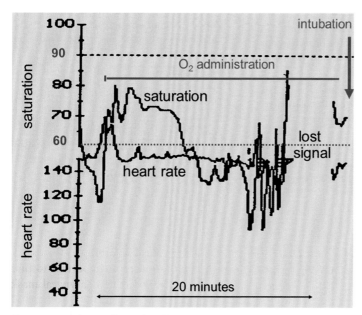

Figure 3.18 A historical recording showing a prolonged period of hypoxia in a child who had undergone adenotonsillectomy because of obstructive sleep apnoea. Pulse oximetry was not yet a routine monitoring device, and was only available for research purposes.

on the history and the presence of large tonsils. Perhaps a more careful observation of the presented child would have raised the suspicion of another or an additional pathology.

Patients who are chronically hypoxic, like children with severe obstructive sleep apnoea, are very sensitive to opioids and probably other sedative drugs (Brown *et al.* 2006). Careful postoperative monitoring is mandatory to prevent severe complications (Coté 2015) (Fig. 3.18).

Summary and Recommendations

Routine preoperative evaluation often supports the more common diagnosis but may miss relevant findings, such as laryngeal stenosis in the presented case.

Translaryngeal jet ventilation via a small catheter may be life-saving, but insufficient expiration leading to barotrauma and cardiovascular collapse is an ever-present threat.

Children with chronic hypoxia are very sensitive to the respiratory depressant action of opioids; careful postoperative monitoring is mandatory.

References

Brown, K.A., Laferriere, A., Lakheeram, I., *et al.* (2006). Recurrent hypoxemia in children is associated with increased analgesic sensitivity to opiates. *Anesthesiology*, 105, 665–669.

Certal, V., Catumbela, E., Winck, J.C., *et al.* (2012). Clinical assessment of pediatric obstructive sleep apnea: a systematic review and meta-analysis. *Laryngoscope*, 122, 2105–2114.

Chan, I.A. & Gamble, J.J. (2016). Tension pneumothorax during flexible bronchoscopy in a nonintubated infant. *Paediatr Anaesth*, 26, 452–454.

Coté, C.J. (2015). Anesthesiological considerations for children with obstructive sleep apnea. *Curr Opin Anaesthesiol*, 28, 327–332.

Duggan, L.V., Ballantyne, S.B., Law, J.A., *et al.* (2016). Transtracheal jet ventilation in the 'can't intubate can't oxygenate' emergency: a systematic review. *Br J Anaesth*, 117 (Suppl. 1), i28–i38.

Gursanscky, J., Boston, M., & Kamani, T. (2017). A snoring child. *BMJ*, 357, j2124.

Hamaekers, A.E., van der Beek, T., Theunissen, M., *et al.* (2015). Rescue ventilation through a small-bore transtracheal cannula in severe hypoxic pigs using expiratory ventilation assistance. *Anesth Analg*, 120, 890–894.

Marcus, C.L., Brooks, L.J., Draper, K.A., *et al.* (2012). Diagnosis and management of childhood obstructive sleep apnea syndrome. *Pediatrics*, 130, e714–e755.

Weiss, M. & Engelhardt, T. (2010). Proposal for the management of the unexpected difficult pediatric airway. *Paediatr Anaesth*, 20, 454–464.

Willemsen, M.G., Noppens, R., Mulder, A.L., *et al.* (2014). Ventilation with the Ventrain through a small lumen catheter in the failed paediatric airway: two case reports. *Br J Anaesth*, 112, 946–947.

Case

Late one evening, a 4-week-old boy, weighing 3940 g, presented with an incarcerated inguinal hernia. The surgeon was able to reduce the hernia, and the boy was scheduled for elective bilateral inguinal hernia repair on the next day. Otherwise, physical examination was unremarkable.

Anaesthesia was uneventful (Fig. 3.19a). After mask induction with sevoflurane and nitrous oxide the airway was secured with a size 1 laryngeal mask airway (LMA) and spontaneous ventilation was maintained during the case. A caudal block was performed and rectal paracetamol was administered. Haemodynamic stability was maintained, oxygen saturation ranged between 95% and 98%, and end-tidal CO_2 was 5.5 kPa.

Postoperatively, the nurses were concerned by a persistent tachypnoea of 60–80 breaths per minute. On the assumption that this could be caused by pain, an additional dose of paracetamol was given and the responsible surgical resident was called. Auscultation of the lungs was normal and there was no need for additional oxygen. Capillary blood gas analysis revealed moderate mixed acidosis with a pH of 7.25, a pCO_2 of 7.34 kPa, and a base excess of –4.4 mmol/l. At this point, a chest x-ray was ordered, which surprisingly showed a left-sided diaphragmatic hernia (Fig. 3.19b).

Two weeks later, the boy underwent uneventful surgical repair of the diaphragmatic hernia. Early extubation could be performed in theatre immediately after surgery.

A delicious detail of this story is that, on admission, a medical student mentioned that he could hear bowel sounds over the left lung. However, a sceptical staff physician repeated lung auscultation and discarded the student's observation.

Discussion

In this patient, a previously unrecognized **congenital diaphragmatic hernia (CDH)** was unmasked by anaesthesia and surgery. During the early few months of life, even significant congenital pathologies may go unnoticed. This time period is characterized by feeding, digesting, sleeping and growing, i.e. activities that do not challenge the cardiovascular or haemostatic systems. Typical examples of pathologies that may be diagnosed late are cardiac anomalies not presenting with cyanosis or severe cardiac failure after birth, e.g. anomalies of the coronary arteries (Heidegger *et al.* 2001), biliary atresia (Hollon *et al.* 2012) or haemophilia, which is usually only diagnosed in the second half of the first year of life (Chambost *et al.* 2002). Before the widespread use of neonatal pulse oximetry screening for cyanotic congenital heart disease (Ewer *et al.* 2012), patients with tetralogy of Fallot may only have been recognized by profound cyanosis when they underwent anaesthesia as an

(a)

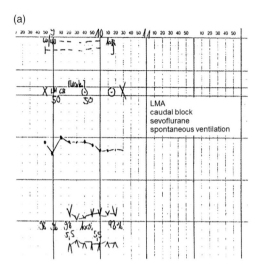

Figure 3.19a The original anaesthesia chart shows an uneventful course with normal oxygen saturation and normal end-tidal CO_2 measurements.

LMA
caudal block
sevoflurane
spontaneous ventilation

(b)

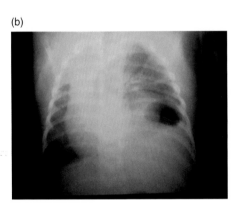

Figure 3.19b The chest x-ray obtained 6 hours after uneventful bilateral inguinal hernia repair showing displacement of the mediastinum to the right.

infant. Later in life, with increasing physical activity, many children become symptomatic, e.g. with dyspnoea or multiple haematomas caused by falls.

The presented case illustrates that preoperative evaluation in the age group 0–6 months is particularly challenging. Even subtle abnormalities may be important. For many institutions, this may be one of the reasons why very young infants are excluded from **outpatient anaesthesia**. It seems to be safer when these very young patients are observed for some time in an inpatient setting. On the other hand, there is no global consensus about the minimal age limit for outpatient anaesthesia. Apart from the arguments mentioned above, there are no stringent arguments to exclude a healthy term neonate from the possibility of same-day discharge after unproblematic anaesthesia and surgery. There is some agreement, however, that prematurely born infants (up to a certain age), children with severe obstructive sleep apnoea, and children with a history of an unexplained life-threatening event should be hospitalized and monitored postoperatively for some time.

CDH usually presents at the time of birth with respiratory failure due to lung hypoplasia and frequently severe pulmonary hypertension. Despite significant advances in intensive care medicine, including sophisticated vasoactive support, the use of selective pulmonary vasodilators and the availability of extracorporeal support (ECMO), mortality rates have remained substantial and prolonged hospital stays are the rule for survivors.

About 20% of infants with CDH belong to a low-risk group with only minimal lung hypoplasia and moderate pulmonary hypertension (Baerg *et al.* 2012). Without prenatal diagnosis, many of these infants adapt normally to extrauterine life. In these patients, the diagnosis is made only after several months or even years, in most cases because of respiratory symptoms that may or may not be related to the CDH leading to an investigation with a chest x-ray. In others, the diagnosis is made because of gastrointestinal symptoms, poor growth or even by chance. Rarely, massive gastric distension leading to cardiac arrest was reported as the primary manifestation (Paut *et al.* 1996). Because the core problems of the disease, lung hypoplasia and pulmonary hypertension, are not predominant, the outcome after adequate treatment is usually very good.

Summary and Recommendations

This case of undiagnosed CDH in a 4-week-old infant scheduled for inguinal hernia repair serves to illustrate that during the first 6 months of life even relevant congenital pathologies may have gone undetected.

CDH usually manifests immediately after birth with severe cardiorespiratory failure. However, about 20% of patients with CDH have no or mild pulmonary hypoplasia and thus fall into a low-risk group. In these patients the diagnosis may be missed at the time of birth.

In addition, the presented case nicely illustrates that careful and attentive nursing observations, followed by a focused workup, can be keys for timely diagnosis.

References

Baerg, J., Kanthimathinathan, V., & Gollin, G. (2012). Late-presenting congenital diaphragmatic hernia: diagnostic pitfalls and outcome. *Hernia*, 16, 461–466.

Chambost, H., Gaboulaud, V., Coatmelec, B., *et al.* (2002). What factors influence the age at diagnosis of hemophilia? Results of the French hemophilia cohort. *J Pediatr*, 141, 548–552.

Ewer, A.K., Furmston, A.T., Middleton, L.J., *et al.* (2012). Pulse oximetry as a screening test for congenital heart defects in newborn infants: a test accuracy study with evaluation of acceptability and cost-effectiveness. *Health Technol Assess*, 16, 1–184.

Heidegger, T., Waidelich, E., & Kreienbuehl, G. (2001). Anomalous origin of the left coronary artery: discovery during an ambulatory surgical procedure in a 3-month old, previously healthy infant. *Paediatr Anaesth*, 11, 109–111.

Hollon, J., Eide, M., & Gorman, G. (2012). Early diagnosis of extrahepatic biliary atresia in an open-access medical system. *PLoS One*, 7, e49643.

Paut, O., Mely, L., Viard, L., *et al.* (1996). Acute presentation of congenital diaphragmatic hernia past the neonatal period: a life threatening emergency. *Can J Anaesth*, 43, 621–625.

Upper Respiratory Tract Infection

Case

Some years ago, an 11-year-old boy, weighing 25 kg, was scheduled for bladder augmentation. The medical history included anal atresia repair, neurogenic bladder dysfunction and moderately reduced renal function. Surgery had already been postponed 2 weeks earlier because of missing capacity in the paediatric intensive care unit (PICU). At the preoperative visit the evening before surgery, he appeared to be in an excellent state of health. The next morning at 7 am, the nurse called the anaesthetist to inform him that there had been occasional coughing during the night and that the body temperature was 38.2 °C. The anaesthetist went to see the patient in his room. He went from the bed to the toilet and back, no coughing was observed, and the oxygen saturation was 95%. In consultation with the parents, it was decided to proceed with surgery.

Anaesthesia was induced with propofol by target-controlled infusion (TCI), remifentanil and mivacurium. Dexmedetomidine was given as a co-analgesic agent in addition to metamizole, dexamethasone and fentanyl. A transverse abdominal plane (TAP) block provided additional analgesia. Vascular access included a radial arterial line and a 14G central venous catheter inserted according to Breschan via the left brachiocephalic vein. More than 6 hours later, immediately after the end of surgery, the patient was extubated. He was pain-free with an oxygen saturation between 93% and 95% while breathing room air.

Over the next 24 hours, a supplemental oxygen requirement and laborious breathing developed. The patient tested positive for rhinovirus. At 60 hours, despite non-invasive treatment with high-flow nasal cannula oxygen, re-intubation was required. The chest x-ray showed a predominantly unilateral opacification (Fig. 3.20). The child was ventilated for 4 days, initially requiring 100% oxygen and a PEEP of 10 cmH$_2$O. This was followed by several days on high-flow nasal oxygen. Finally, the patient left hospital on the 18th postoperative day.

Discussion

The case history of this child, who developed symptoms of a **mild upper respiratory tract infection (URTI)** on the day he was scheduled to undergo major surgery, illustrates that nothing should be taken for granted in clinical medicine. URTIs are common in children, with 4–6 annual episodes over the first few years of life (Heikkinen & Jarvinen 2003). In the winter season, every fourth child has a cold at any given time point, and almost half of all children have a history of an URTI within the last 6 weeks (Parnis *et al.* 2001). Therefore, postponing surgery in all children with mild colds is not a realistic option. Although acute airway complications, such as laryngospasm, coughing or stridor, are more common in

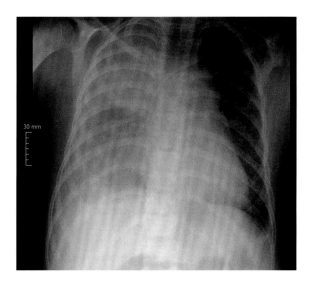

Figure 3.20 Chest x-ray taken prior to re-intubation on the third postoperative day. On the day of major abdominal surgery, this child had developed mild symptoms of a common cold.

these children, it is generally agreed that these complications can be anticipated, easily recognized and adequately treated by a skilled anaesthetist (Tait & Malviya 2005). Even in open heart surgery, no increase in mortality has been reported for such children (Malviya *et al.* 2003). In the context of the presented case, it is nevertheless noteworthy that there was an increased incidence of atelectasis in the same case series. Many anaesthetists would accept a child for anaesthesia who is in a good state of health, with occasional coughing, normal oxygen saturation and a body temperature below 38.5 °C. Indeed, with this practice, the perioperative course will be uneventful in most cases.

Rhinovirus is a common cause of URTI in children. In a few patients, however, pneumonia or even acute respiratory distress syndrome can develop (Soni *et al.* 2017). In paediatric cardiac surgery, rhinovirus infection is related to extubation failure and prolonged hospital stay (Delgado-Corcoran *et al.* 2014). In the presented case, one could speculate that the protracted postoperative course was also influenced by fluid overload in the presence of an impaired renal function and inadequate positioning with the affected lung down (Fig. 3.20). The key question is if the complicated postoperative course could have been anticipated in this patient. But even in hindsight, the answer is probably no.

Preoperative inhalation with a beta-stimulating agent has been recommended for the **prevention** of acute airway complications in children with URTIs (von Ungern-Sternberg *et al.* 2009); in contrast, the value of anticholinergic medication at induction is debatable (Tait *et al.* 2007). At least in infants, pre-treatment with oral atropine seems to reduce airway-related complications (Shaw *et al.* 2000). If surgery is postponed, 2 weeks seems to be sufficient to reduce the risk (von Ungern-Sternberg *et al.* 2010). It is best to avoid airway instrumentation or at least endotracheal intubation.

Summary and Recommendations

Critical respiratory events, such as laryngospasm, bronchospasm, coughing and desaturation, are more common in children with URTIs.

The skilled anaesthetist, however, will almost always be able to anticipate, readily recognize and successfully treat these complications.

Nothing can be taken for granted in clinical medicine. This case illustrates that, occasionally, even a common cold can lead to severe and protracted postoperative pulmonary morbidity.

References

Delgado-Corcoran, C., Witte, M.K., Ampofo, K., *et al.* (2014). The impact of human rhinovirus infection in pediatric patients undergoing heart surgery. *Pediatr Cardiol,* 35, 1387–1394.

Heikkinen, T. & Jarvinen, A. (2003). The common cold. *Lancet,* 361, 51–59.

Malviya, S., Voepel-Lewis, T., Siewert, M., *et al.* (2003). Risk factors for adverse postoperative outcomes in children presenting for cardiac surgery with upper respiratory tract infections. *Anesthesiology,* 98, 628–632.

Parnis, S.J., Barker, D.S., & van der Walt, J.H. (2001). Clinical predictors of anaesthetic complications in children with respiratory tract infections. *Paediatr Anaesth,* 11, 29–40.

Shaw, C.A., Kelleher, A.A., Gill, C.P., *et al.* (2000). Comparison of the incidence of complications at induction and emergence in infants receiving oral atropine vs no premedication. *Br J Anaesth,* 84, 174–178.

Soni, P., Rai, A., Aggarwal, N., *et al.* (2017). Enterovirus-human rhinovirus: a rare cause of acute respiratory distress syndrome. *J Investig Med High Impact Case Rep,* 5, 2324709617728526.

Tait, A.R., Burke, C., Voepel-Lewis, T., *et al.* (2007). Glycopyrrolate does not reduce the incidence of perioperative adverse events in children with upper respiratory tract infections. *Anesth Analg,* 104, 265–270.

Tait, A.R. & Malviya, S. (2005). Anesthesia for the child with an upper respiratory tract infection: still a dilemma? *Anesth Analg,* 100, 59–65.

von Ungern-Sternberg, B.S., Boda, K., Chambers, N.A., *et al.* (2010). Risk assessment for respiratory complications in paediatric anaesthesia: a prospective cohort study. *Lancet,* 376, 773–783.

von Ungern-Sternberg, B.S., Habre, W., Erb, T.O., *et al.* (2009). Salbutamol premedication in children with a recent respiratory tract infection. *Paediatr Anaesth,* 19, 1064–1069.

4 Vascular Access

Difficult Venous Access

Case

Several decades ago, a 2 6/12-year-old girl was transferred to the children's hospital because of severe dehydration and shock following gastroenteritis. Numerous attempts to obtain venous access were unsuccessful, and the anaesthesia team was called for help. The anaesthetist inserted an intraosseous Cook cannula into the right proximal tibia. Fluid resuscitation was performed, and some hours later a peripheral venous cannula was successfully placed. The decision was taken to leave the intraosseous needle in place for the following 48 hours to have a back-up in case of loss of peripheral venous access. The girl recovered and left hospital.

Six weeks later, she was readmitted and diagnosed with osteomyelitis of the right proximal tibia, the exact same site where the intraosseous cannula had previously been placed. The site was surgically drained. From the pus enteritic salmonella were cultured, the same organism found in stool and blood cultures during the first hospitalization.

Discussion

The presented case of **osteomyelitis** after **intraosseous cannulation** reminds us that this clearly beneficial and often life-saving technique can have potentially significant complications (Neuhaus 2014). It is very likely that local tissue damage caused by the cannula in the spongiosa enhanced adherence of bacteria during bacteraemia. In retrospect, the intraosseous needle was unnecessarily left in place for a prolonged period. It seems advisable to remove an intraosseous needle as early as possible, i.e. immediately after venous access has been obtained, or after 24 hours at the latest, to minimize risks of infection. Following this case, it has been the author's practice to administer a single dose of an antibiotic, e.g. cefuroxime, in the rare cases when intraosseous needles had been placed.

Complications do occur after intraosseous cannulation. In a large Scandinavian series, including 1802 cases, the following complication rates were reported: dislocation (8.5%), extravasation (3.7%), compartment syndrome (0.6%) and osteomyelitis (0.4%) (Hallas *et al.* 2013). In addition, bone fractures (La Fleche *et al.* 1989) and broken needles (Hallas *et al.* 2013) have been reported. The author has encountered a circular skin burn caused by the EZ-IO system: a needle was used that was too short because of marked tissue swelling secondary to the administration of local anaesthetic (Fig. 4.1). The most serious complication is extravasation leading to compartment syndrome; in some cases, this has even resulted in the loss of an extremity (Suominen *et al.* 2015). Therefore, it is of paramount importance to continuously observe the area of needle insertion in order to be able to stop

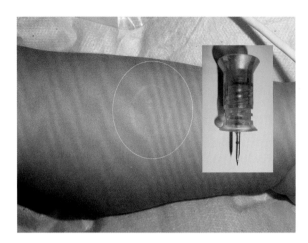

Figure 4.1 Circular scar caused by an intraosseous needle.

fluid administration immediately when swelling occurs (Dasgupta & Playfor 2010). This can easily be done during resuscitation, but may be difficult during surgery, when the legs may not be accessible.

The EZ-IO system, an easy-to-use drill-assisted device, is the most popular product used today (Hafner *et al.* 2013). When dedicated material is not available, a normal 18G intravenous cannula can be used (Hamed *et al.* 2013). In children, the proximal tibia is the insertion site preferred by most practitioners, followed by the distal tibia or the distal femur.

An **indication** for intraosseous access is clearly given for resuscitation when peripheral venous cannulation is not immediately successful. Most clinicians will even directly proceed to intraosseous cannulation, when a rapid successful peripheral venous puncture seems unlikely. In contrast, there is an ongoing debate regarding the **semi-elective use** of intraosseous cannulation for anaesthesia in cases of difficult venous access (Neuhaus *et al.* 2010). The author has used this approach a few times in severely ill children for fluid administration and anaesthesia induction until central or peripheral venous catheterization was successful.

In cases of **difficult venous access** during elective anaesthesia, however, most clinicians will rely on an ultrasound-guided puncture, e.g. of the cephalic vein on the forearm, which is highly successful in experienced hands in the anaesthetized non-moving child. Alternatively, deep veins such as the femoral, internal jugular, brachiocephalic or subclavian vein can be cannulated. In exceptional cases, experienced anaesthetists occasionally proceed with anaesthesia for short (Jöhr & Can 1993) or non-invasive procedures (Wilson & Engelhardt 2012) without an intravenous access.

Summary and Recommendations

Intraosseous cannulation is an important technique in emergency medicine and, in a few exceptional cases, for the care of severely ill children in the operating theatre.

Intraosseous access should be removed as early as possible in order to minimize the risk of extravasation, compartment syndrome and infectious complications.

References

Dasgupta, S. & Playfor, S.D. (2010). Intraosseous fluid resuscitation in meningococcal disease and lower limb injury. *Pediatr Rep*, 2 (1), e5.

Hafner, J.W., Bryant, A., Huang, F., *et al.* (2013). Effectiveness of a drill-assisted intraosseous catheter versus manual intraosseous catheter by resident physicians in a swine model. *West J Emerg Med*, 14, 629–632.

Hallas, P., Brabrand, M., & Folkestad, L. (2013). Complication with intraosseous access: Scandinavian users' experience. *West J Emerg Med*, 14, 440–443.

Hamed, R.K., Hartmans, S., & Gausche-Hill, M. (2013). Anesthesia through an intraosseous line using an 18-gauge intravenous needle for emergency pediatric surgery. *J Clin Anesth*, 25, 447–451.

Jöhr, M. & Can, U. (1993). Pediatric anesthesia without vascular access: intramuscular administration of atracurium. *Anesth Analg*, 76, 1162–1163.

La Fleche, F.R., Slepin, M.J., Vargas, J., *et al.* (1989). Iatrogenic bilateral tibial fractures after intraosseous infusion attempts in a 3-month-old infant. *Ann Emerg Med*, 18, 1099–1101.

Neuhaus, D. (2014). Intraosseous infusion in elective and emergency pediatric anesthesia: when should we use it? *Curr Opin Anaesthesiol*, 27, 282–287.

Neuhaus, D., Weiss, M., Engelhardt, T., *et al.* (2010). Semi-elective intraosseous infusion after failed intravenous access in pediatric anesthesia. *Paediatr Anaesth*, 20, 168–171.

Suominen, P.K., Nurmi, E., & Lauerma, K. (2015). Intraosseous access in neonates and infants: risk of severe complications: a case report. *Acta Anaesthesiol Scand*, 59, 1389–1393.

Wilson, G. & Engelhardt, T. (2012). Who needs an IV? Retrospective service analysis in a tertiary pediatric hospital. *Paediatr Anaesth*, 22, 442–444.

Extravasation

Case

A long time ago, a girl born at 38 weeks of gestation with a birth weight of 2500 g was scheduled for the repair of a left-sided diaphragmatic hernia on day of life 5. She was nasotracheally intubated and on conventional ventilation with an FiO_2 of 0.21. When she arrived in the operating theatre, an umbilical arterial catheter (UAC), a peripherally inserted 27G central venous catheter (PICC) and a closed 24G catheter (Insyte) on the left foot were in place. After careful evaluation, a decision was made to use these devices during the case. It was reported that the peripheral venous catheter was functioning well and only closed some minutes ago for transfer to the theatre. In addition, the line was rapidly flushed with 5 ml of normal saline without adverse events.

The anaesthetic management included a bolus of thiopental, sevoflurane and a continuous infusion of mivacurium; in addition, a caudal block with ropivacaine and morphine was performed. The PICC was used for the continuous administration of medications and glucose, whereas crystalloids and colloids were infused via the peripheral venous line. By the end of the 3-hour case, 30 ml hydroxyethyl starch, 40 ml of a balanced crystalloid solution (Ringerfundin) and a 6 ml bolus of an antibiotic had been given. The peripheral line was flushed with normal saline with the intention to close it again for transfer. When the drapes were removed, massive swelling of the foot with blister formation was seen (Fig. 4.2a). The blister was removed by the surgeon and the foot was aseptically dressed.

The postoperative course was uneventful and the girl was extubated on postoperative day 3. Fortunately, the extravasation did not result in ischaemia or deep tissue necrosis. Nevertheless, the patient had to return repeatedly to the operating theatre for debridement and dressing changes.

Discussion

Infiltration of a venous line is an ever-present threat. Even when the catheter tip has a perfect intravascular position at the beginning of the case, fluid can leak along the catheter into the subcutaneous tissue, especially when high pressures are applied and the venous flow is impaired by thrombus formation. Over time, incremental swelling can cause the catheter to be pulled out. Even if the correct position is verified by flushing and by ultrasound (Gautam *et al.* 2017), there is no guarantee that late displacement, as described in this case, will not occur. When a line has just been inserted and a long segment of it is in an intravascular position, one can be confident that it will stay in place. However, many of these venous catheters are only 15–18 mm long, and only a few millimetres are placed within the vessel. Sometimes, replacing such a short catheter immediately after insertion by

(a)

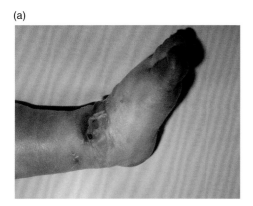

Figure 4.2a This extravasation was visible after the removal of the drapes. The infusion was administered through an initially well-running 24G cannula in the great saphenous vein.

a longer one via a 0.018 inch guidewire is an option. Following this case, for major neonatal surgery the author mostly used venous catheters that had been newly inserted under his supervision, at least when intraoperative access to the access site was not possible. Alternatively, particularly when massive volume shifts were expected during neonatal surgery, he preferred to insert a central venous catheter into the internal jugular vein, e.g. a 4F double-lumen catheter.

When vasoactive drugs are infused over peripheral lines, massive local vasoconstriction impeding venous drainage seems to increase the risk of infiltration; nevertheless the administration of vasoactive compounds, especially dopamine, over a restricted time period using a peripheral line is common practice with a low morbidity (Patregnani *et al.* 2017).

On the ward, **prevention** of extravasation consists in a regular inspection of the infusion site (Tofani *et al.* 2012), as well as in setting the pressure alarm of the infusion pump at a very low level. It is noteworthy that even with an umbilical venous catheter that is not in the desired ideal position, extravasation can occur (Hollingsworth *et al.* 2015). Among all superficial veins, the external jugular vein is probably the one most prone to dislodgement, leading to extravasation into the loose neck tissue. For this reason, it was the author's practice never to use an external jugular venous catheter for postoperative intravenous therapy. Even when the drip is running spontaneously, the tip of the cannula could be in the extravascular space.

Treatment of extravasation mainly consists in avoiding additional damage. Sometimes, especially in acute cases like the one described here, a proportion of the fluid can be squeezed out through the entry hole of the cannula, allowing rapid reduction of tissue pressure. Accidental subfascial infusion can lead to a compartment syndrome requiring fasciotomy (Fig. 4.2b) (Pasquesoone *et al.* 2016). When necrotic lesions are observed, it is wise to wait until they become clearly delineated. If only crystalloids, artificial colloids or blood products and no toxic compounds have been administered, prognosis is usually good. However, there are no evidence-based recommendations for the management of extravasations (Reynolds *et al.* 2014).

Every undesired event should be communicated to the parents as early as possible. In the presented case, in line with his usual practice, the anaesthetist had spoken with the parents every 90 minutes over the phone to inform them of the progress of surgery and any potential problems during anaesthesia. They were understanding and forgiving, and even comforted the frustrated anaesthetist.

(b)

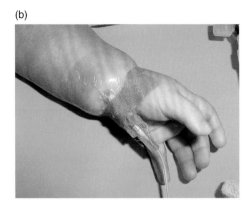

Figure 4.2b This extravasation caused ischaemia of the hand. Some of the fluid could be squeezed out through the entry hole of the cannula, and the hand subsequently turned pink.

Summary and Recommendations

The case presented here shows that extravasation is an ever-present threat, even when the venous catheter was initially in a correct intravascular position.

The site of venous access should be monitored regularly; if this is not feasible, e.g. during surgery, it may be wise to insert a new device, and to select one which can be inserted into the vein over a long distance.

References

Gautam, N.K., Bober, K.R., & Cai, C. (2017). Introduction of color-flow injection test to confirm intravascular location of peripherally placed intravenous catheters. *Paediatr Anaesth*, 27, 821–826.

Hollingsworth, C., Clarke, P., Sharma, A., *et al.* (2015). National survey of umbilical venous catheterisation practices in the wake of two deaths. *Arch Dis Child Fetal Neonatal Ed*, 100, F371–F372.

Pasquesoone, L., Aljudaibi, N., Ellart, J., *et al.* (2016). Emergency management of extravasation in children [in French]. *Ann Chir Plast Esthet*, 61, 598–604.

Patregnani, J.T., Sochet, A.A., & Klugman, D. (2017). Short-term peripheral vasoactive infusions in pediatrics: where is the harm? *Pediatr Crit Care Med*, 18, e378–e381.

Reynolds, P.M., MacLaren, R., Mueller, S.W., *et al.* (2014). Management of extravasation injuries: a focused evaluation of noncytotoxic medications. *Pharmacotherapy*, 34, 617–632.

Tofani, B.F., Rineair, S.A., Gosdin, C.H., *et al.* (2012). Quality improvement project to reduce infiltration and extravasation events in a pediatric hospital. *J Pediatr Nurs*, 27, 682–689.

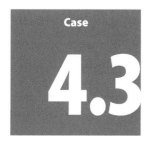

Case

4.3

Paravenous Drug Injection

Case

A long time ago, a 9-year-old girl, weighing 30 kg, sustained a femoral fracture in a skiing accident. On the scene, paramedics established intravenous access in the right cubital fossa, administered fentanyl 50 μg and midazolam 2.5 mg, followed by a Ringer's lactate drip. She was transported first by rescue sledge and then by ambulance over 60 km to the paediatric hospital. After an x-ray had been taken, the girl was brought directly to theatre for closed reduction and internal fixation of her femur. She was still on the initial emergency stretcher wearing her padded ski suit.

The anaesthetic plan included intravenous induction, endotracheal intubation and a femoral nerve block for postoperative analgesia. Proper functioning of the venous line was verified by the injection of fentanyl 50 μg flushed in with 10 ml of normal saline. Ringer's lactate was dripping freely by gravity alone, leaving only a small remainder in the bag.

Anaesthesia was induced by injections of thiopental 2.5% 175 mg and succinylcholine 50 mg. Both were forcefully flushed in with 10 ml of normal saline. We wished her a good sleep and, well behaved, she closed her eyes. Cricoid pressure was applied. About 30 seconds later, she opened her eyes and asked 'Why are you pressing on my throat?'

The suspected course of events soon became clear when the padded ski suit was retracted, exposing a massively swollen right elbow. Rapidly, venous access was established on the opposite hand and additional doses of thiopental and succinylcholine were injected intravenously. The further anaesthetic course was uneventful.

Discussion

This case of **paravenous injection** of thiopental and succinylcholine prompts consideration of two issues: first, the unrecognized malposition of a venous cannula, and second, the potential tissue toxicity of injected compounds.

Every effort should be made to **ensure the correct intravenous position** of a cannula before it is used for induction. This includes flushing without resistance and pain (done in the presented case), and inspection of the cannula site (not done in the presented case). Even an infusion dripping freely by gravity does not reliably prove correct cannula placement, especially in regions with loose subcutaneous tissue, e.g. at the neck or, as in this case, the cubital fossa. Undoubtedly, inspection of the cannula site during flushing would have avoided the complication. The author has to admit that in daily practice, especially when infants and young children are not cooperative upon arrival to the theatre, he often uses an existing intravenous access and does not always remove the bandages and the splint to inspect the cannula site. Ultrasound is increasingly used to verify that injected fluid can be seen in a venous vessel (Gautam *et al.* 2017).

Subcutaneously injected drugs will be absorbed and can cause clinical effects. While sedation by the hypnotic agent may be desirable, the onset of paralysis caused by subcutaneously injected succinylcholine would be a disaster for the child. In this case, 1.7 mg/kg of succinylcholine was given, less than the dose required for complete paralysis after intramuscular injection (Schuh 1982); nevertheless it is wise in such cases to induce general anaesthesia as rapidly as possible.

Paravenous injection can **cause tissue damage** (Le & Patel 2014). It has been known for a long time that subcutaneously injected thiopental can lead to tissue necrosis (Davies 1966). Solutions with lower concentrations, e.g. thiopental 1% or 2.5%, are less disastrous than the classical 5% solution. Indeed, the author has never encountered relevant tissue damage during his career (spanning 40 years in clinical anaesthesia), despite a number of accidental subcutaneous injections of 1% or 2.5% solutions of thiopental. Nevertheless, it is probably wise to use the less toxic propofol instead of thiopental if there is the slightest doubt about the proper positioning of a venous line. In the author's experience, ketamine may be a good option in toddlers, because it will rapidly calm the situation to allow inspection of the venous access site. The most common cause of tissue necrosis following paravenous injection involves calcium-containing solutions; the author remembers several such cases, especially in neonates (Fig. 4.3).

Another reason why thiopental should not be injected through a cannula lying in the cubital fossa is the possibility of unrecognized **intra-arterial injection** (cf. Case 4.4), which can lead to catastrophic complications including gangrene and limb amputation (Khan & Noorbaksh 2004, Kinmonth & Sheperd 1959). It seems wise to never inject thiopental into a catheter lying in the cubital fossa.

Summary and Recommendations

The described case of accidental paravenous injection of thiopental and succinylcholine in a 9-year-old girl shows a complication that appears completely avoidable (at least when judged in retrospect from the writing desk).

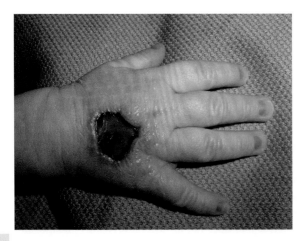

Figure 4.3 Skin necrosis after extravasation of calcium gluconate in a neonate.

Both local toxicity and absorption, with ensuing clinical effects, have to be considered after paravenous injection.

The case also nicely illustrates that performing only some parts of a safety checklist is not enough. A venous line must be dripping freely and easily flushable without causing any discomfort; in addition, inspection of the cannula site should raise no concerns.

The delicious irony of the presented story is that the author did not follow the rule to 'never inject thiopental into a vein in the cubital fossa', a rule that he had himself established in his institution.

References

Davies, D.D. 1966. Local complications of thiopentone injection. *Br J Anaesth*, 38, 530–532.

Gautam, N.K., Bober, K.R., & Cai, C. (2017). Introduction of color-flow injection test to confirm intravascular location of peripherally placed intravenous catheters. *Paediatr Anaesth*, 27, 821–826.

Khan, Z.H. & Noorbaksh, S. (2004). An accidental intra-arterial injection of thiopental on the dorsum of the foot: a case report. *Acta Anaesthesiol.Taiwan*, 42, 55–58.

Kinmonth, J.B. & Sheperd, R.C. (1959). Accidental injection of thiopentone into arteries: studies of pathology and treatment. *Br Med J*, 2 (5157), 914–918.

Le, A. & Patel, S. (2014). Extravasation of noncytotoxic drugs: a review of the literature. *Ann Pharmacother*, 48, 870–886.

Schuh, F.T. (1982). The neuromuscular blocking action of suxamethonium following intravenous and intramuscular administration. *Int J Clin Pharmacol Ther Toxicol*, 20, 399–403.

Intra-Arterial Injection

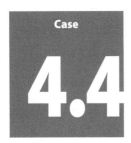

Case

Many years ago, a 2-month-old boy, weighing 4 kg, was scheduled for inguinal hernia repair. After inhalational induction, the airway was secured with a size 1 classic type laryngeal mask airway (LMA). Venous access proved to be difficult, leading to attempts on the scalp. Finally, a 26G Abbocath was successfully inserted into a vessel. There was only moderate backflow of blood; however, when the line was flushed with normal saline, a wide skin area immediately blanched (Fig. 4.4). Intra-arterial position was assumed and the catheter was removed before any active compounds had been injected.

Discussion

In the presented case, inadvertent **intra-arterial placement of the cannula** was recognized in time. Intra-arterial placement of peripheral catheters typically occurs on the scalp, in the antecubital fossa and at the radial aspect of the distal forearm. On the head, skin blanching can readily be recognized when the line is flushed. At all other sites, this is not the case and a high index of suspicion is required. Numerous cases of accidental intra-arterial injections have been reported in adults (Ghouri *et al.* 2002) and in children (Duggan & Braude 2004), most of them involving the use of thiopental and some of propofol. Whereas thiopental is directly toxic to the vascular endothelium (MacPherson *et al.* 1991), propofol is not (MacPherson *et al.* 1992). With propofol, except for one case (Ang 1998), only transient erythema but no long-term consequences have been reported. Intra-arterial injection of atracurium can lead to vasospasm (Kessell & Barker 1996) or no visible reaction (as described below).

In some children, usually with an extensive past medical history, venous access can be very difficult and only a very thin vein can be cannulated, e.g. on the back of the hand or on the palmar surface of the distal forearm. In such cases, there can be marked resistance to injection and blanching of the skin because venous drainage is limited and injected fluid is flooding back into the capillary system. It can thus be difficult to determine the correct position of such lines. Such cannulas should only be used very cautiously and replaced as early as possible.

A previously placed **arterial line** can erroneously be used to inject drugs. In his professional career, the author has made this painful error on two occasions in adults, once injecting midazolam and once injecting atracurium, fortunately with no long-term consequences. Colour-coding of the three-way stopcocks is helpful to avoid such errors, and it may be wise to additionally protect the injection port of an arterial line by applying a tape.

In some desperate cases, it might be tempting to use an existing arterial line to administer drugs. In neonatology, a large variety of compounds have been given via an umbilical

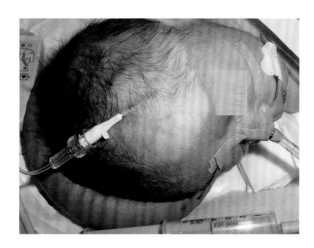

Figure 4.4 Typical intra-arterial placement of a cannula with blanching of the skin following flushing (from Jöhr, M. (2017). Complications in paediatric anaesthesia. *Anästh Intensivmed*, 58, 259–266, with permission).

artery catheter without obvious negative consequences. This can probably be explained by the fact that the injection is made into the aorta, with a very high blood flow and rapid drug dilution; when a peripheral artery is used, this is not the case. In anaesthesia, the only generally accepted drugs for intra-arterial use are heparin (to keep the line open) and local anaesthetics (Koscielniak-Nielsen & Horn 1993). Because of the paucity of available safety data, voluntary intra-arterial administration of any drug should probably be avoided.

Once intra-arterial injections have occurred, evidence-based **treatments** are largely lacking (Crawford & Terranova 1990). It seems reasonable to use heparin to prevent further thrombosis and to maintain sufficient perfusion pressure. The use of sympatholytic blocks has been reported (Kessell & Barker 1996).

Summary and Recommendations

Even in expert hands, intra-arterial cannula placement occasionally occurs when venous access is attempted. Timely recognition of cannula misplacement is of paramount importance.

Whenever there is the slightest doubt, a non-toxic compound should be chosen, e.g. propofol instead of thiopental. Remember: 'Never inject thiopental into an elbow vein.'

Colour-coding of three-way stopcocks and even taping the injection port can help to prevent its inadvertent use for drug administration.

References

Ang, B.L. (1998). Prolonged cutaneous sequelae after intra-arterial injection of propofol. *Singapore Med J*, 39, 124–126.

Crawford, C.R. & Terranova, W.A. (1990). The role of intraarterial vasodilators in the treatment of inadvertent intraarterial injection injuries. *Ann Plast Surg*, 25, 279–282.

Duggan, M. & Braude, B.M. (2004). Accidental intra-arterial injection through an 'intravenous' cannula on the dorsum of the hand. *Paediatr Anaesth*, 14, 611–612.

Ghouri, A.F., Mading, W., & Prabaker, K. (2002). Accidental intraarterial drug injections via intravascular catheters placed on the dorsum of the hand. *Anesth Analg*, 95, 487–491.

Kessell, G. & Barker, I. (1996). Leg ischaemia in an infant following accidental intra-arterial administration of atracurium treated with caudal anaesthesia. *Anaesthesia*, 51, 1154–1156.

Koscielniak-Nielsen, Z.J. & Horn, A. (1993). Intra-arterial versus intravenous regional analgesia for hand surgery. *Anaesthesia*, 48, 769–772.

MacPherson, R.D., McLeod, L.J., & Grove, A.J. (1991). Intra-arterial thiopentone is directly toxic to vascular endothelium. *Br J Anaesth*, 67, 546–552.

MacPherson, R.D., Rasiah, R.L., & McLeod, L.J. (1992). Intraarterial propofol is not directly toxic to vascular endothelium. *Anesthesiology*, 76, 967–971.

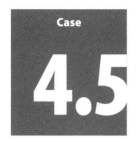

Case

4.5

The Three-Way Stopcock Phenomenon

Case

A 4-week-old infant, weighing 3.6 kg, was scheduled for open pyloromyotomy. Following the administration of thiopental 7 mg/kg and atracurium 0.55 mg/kg, the trachea was intubated with an oral uncuffed endotracheal tube size 3.5. Anaesthesia was maintained with halothane, nitrous oxide and an additional dose of atracurium 0.27 mg/kg just prior to skin incision. For postoperative analgesia, a caudal block with bupivacaine 0.125% 2 ml/kg with adrenaline was placed and rectal paracetamol was administered.

One hour after induction, 40 minutes after skin incision, neuromuscular monitoring showed full recovery with four equal responses after train-of-four (TOF) stimulation. The infant was extubated while fully awake and spontaneously breathing. After monitoring the infant for 10 more minutes, transfer to the ward was initiated. When the nurse from the ward arrived, a rapidly decreasing oxygen saturation was noted and the infant was found to be cyanotic, completely flaccid and with gasping respiratory efforts. Bag-mask ventilation rapidly restored oxygen saturation, but the baby continued to have only minimal muscle tone.

Analysis of the events rapidly led to the correct diagnosis: at the time of arrival of the nurse from the ward, the intravenous line was flushed through the three-way stopcock to confirm patency. The female hub still contained atracurium, the last drug administered during anaesthesia. This was confirmed by neuromuscular monitoring showing massive fading after TOF stimulation. Administration of neostigmine and atropine rapidly restored normal muscle tone and respiration pattern.

Discussion

This case illustrates the importance of flushing intravenous lines and especially **three-way stopcocks** (Fig. 4.5a) in order to avoid **inadvertent administration of residual drugs** (Bowman *et al.* 2013). This is particularly relevant when neuromuscular blocking agents are flushed into small children, as in this case. With the exception of the injection of remifentanil, which causes visible rigor and significant bradycardia, the clinical signs with other drugs may be more subtle. The consequences of a small dose of a neuromuscular blocking agent become less dramatic in older children. However, in view of the 'iceberg phenomenon', which means that at the time of full clinical recovery a large portion of acetylcholine receptors still remain blocked and the margin of safety of the neuromuscular transmission is greatly reduced (Waud & Waud 1971), the three-way stopcock phenomenon can be a relevant problem in older children as well (Fig. 4.5b). Some clinicians may use such an event to argue for routine reversal after the administration of a

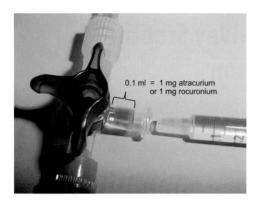

0.1 ml = 1 mg atracurium
or 1 mg rocuronium

Figure 4.5a The female hub contains 0.1 ml, which equals 1 mg rocuronium or atracurium. This dose (0.3 mg/kg) is equivalent to the administration of ED_{95} to a 3 kg baby.

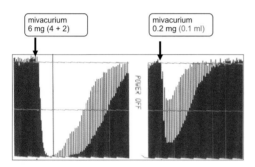

mivacurium
6 mg (4 + 2)

mivacurium
0.2 mg (0.1 ml)

Figure 4.5b This graph illustrates the time course of neuromuscular blockade after the administration of mivacurium 6 mg (0.2 mg/kg) to a child weighing 31 kg. At the time of full recovery, with no visible fading after TOF stimulation, a small dose of 0.2 mg (0.1 ml) leads to relevant neuromuscular block, because many of the receptors are still occupied by the curare molecule.

non-depolarizing neuromuscular blocking agent, so that the relaxant is never the last drug in the intravenous line and the margin of safety of the neuromuscular transmission might be increased. However, such a stringent and non-individualized approach was not the author's practice.

This case also emphasizes that it is not only the dead space of intravenous tubing or portacath systems (Ben-Arush & Berant 1996) that can cause problems, but also a small volume such as in the hub of a three-way stopcock, where the female hub contains 0.1 ml and the male hub 0.05 ml; these dead-space volumes should be considered during the administration of drugs dissolved in a small volume, e.g. during neonatal anaesthesia.

This complication of a three-way stopcock phenomenon was not trivial. While no harm occurred to this patient, because apnoea was immediately recognized and treated, the same 'routine flushing' of an intravenous line on the ward, with less skilled personnel, might have led to a completely different outcome.

Several cases of inadvertent administration of residual drugs have been reported in the literature (Davidson & Brown 1996, Khan et al. 2002) and the problem should be known to the anaesthesia community. Surprisingly, however, this seems not to be the case, and the entity was described as a new phenomenon decades after the presented case (Hoesni et al. 2010).

Drugs have to be flushed in. It is a good practice to always use the same hub and dedicated syringes filled with normal saline for flushing, e.g. during the sequence 'hypnotic–saline–relaxant–saline', and not simply to turn the running drip higher.

Summary and Recommendations

This case emphasizes the need to always flush the line after the administration of drugs to free the system (including three-way stopcocks) of residual amounts of the compound, to avoid potentially severe harm.

The discussion about the inadvertent administration of residual drugs also shows that practitioners are often not aware of published knowledge. This emphasizes the importance of reading and taking advantage of the experience of the past.

References

Ben-Arush, M. & Berant, M. (1996). Retention of drugs in venous access port chamber: a note of caution. *BMJ*, 312, 496–497.

Bowman, S., Raghavan, K., & Walker, I.A. (2013). Residual anaesthesia drugs in intravenous lines: a silent threat? *Anaesthesia*, 68, 557–561.

Davidson, A. & Brown, T.C. (1996). Respiratory arrest in two children following postoperative flushing of suxamethonium from the deadspace of intravenous cannulae. *Anaesth Intensive Care*, 24, 97–98.

Hoesni, S., Tan, K., & Crowe, S. (2010). Inadvertent administration of drug residue causing respiratory arrest: case series. *Eur J Anaesthesiol*, 27, 846–848.

Khan, R.I., Khan, F.H., & Naqvi, H.I. (2002). Respiratory arrest in a child after flushing of pancuronium from the deadspace of intravenous cannula. *J Pak Med Assoc*, 52, 487–488.

Waud, B.E. & Waud, D.R. (1971). The relation between tetanic fade and receptor occlusion in the presence of competitive neuromuscular block. *Anesthesiology*, 35, 456–464.

Vascular Damage

Case

Many years ago, long before the arrival of ultrasound into paediatric anaesthesia practice, a 6-month-old girl, weighing 7 kg, was scheduled for the resection of an ossified cephalohaematoma. Anaesthesia was induced by mask with sevoflurane and nitrous oxide. Peripheral venous access was difficult, and despite multiple attempts ultimately unsuccessful. Femoral venous access was attempted on both sides, puncturing with a 22G steel cannula; blood could be aspirated repeatedly, but the insertion of the guidewire was unsuccessful. During the attempts on the right side, red, potentially arterial blood had been seen a few times in the hub of the needle.

When the drapes were removed, a completely white right leg was apparent. Pedal pulses were not palpable and the pulse oximeter signal was absent (Fig. 4.6a and 4.6b). In the left groin, after a further attempt, the insertion of a 3F central venous catheter was finally successful. As no improvement occurred over the next few minutes the decision was made to perform a caudal block with 8 ml bupivacaine 0.125% with adrenaline for sympathicolysis. About 30 minutes later a pulse oximeter signal became detectable; the leg was still pale, but the team ventured to proceed with surgery. At the end of the case the leg appeared normal, with palpable pedal pulses (Fig. 4.6c).

Discussion

This case illustrates that multiple attempts at vascular cannulation are not without harm and can cause **vascular damage** (Bodenham *et al.* 2016). In this case probably multiple lacerations of the femoral artery led to profound vasospasm and so caused leg ischaemia. However, at first glance, arterial dissection and thrombosis or even an interrupted continuity can initially never be ruled out. If ischaemia had persisted, a duplex sonographic examination followed by vascular surgical advice would have been needed. The author has heard of cases where a surgical revision was needed, but he has never seen one personally. The problem is obviously much more serious when the cardiologists insert larger catheters (Lin *et al.* 2001). Based on this case with leg ischaemia, it became the author's practice to initiate prophylactic medication with tranexamic acid, well established for cranioplasty surgery (Goobie *et al.* 2017), only after the successful vascular cannulations in order to preserve some fibrinolytic potential in case of distal ischaemia.

After arterial damage, absent perfusion, as in this case, or a severe haemorrhage can occur. As a rule of thumb, the simple puncture of most structures with a 24G plastic cannula (e.g. Insyte) is usually not followed by serious consequences, as long as no guidewire is inserted and dilatation is performed. The **'real weapon'** of the anaesthetist is

(a)

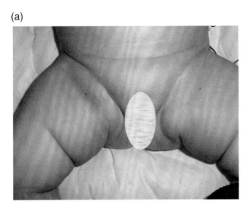

Figure 4.6a Unsuccessful inguinal venous punctures resulting in an ischaemic right lower leg after multiple inadvertent punctures of the right femoral artery.

(b)

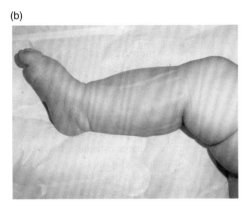

Figure 4.6b Ischaemic right lower leg with absent pedal pulses.

(c)

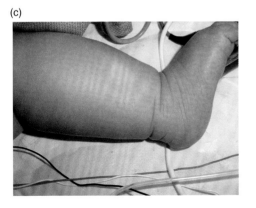

Figure 4.6c Normal appearance of the leg at the end of the case.

dilatation. Before it is performed the practitioner has to be absolutely sure that the guide-wire is in the lumen of the desired venous vessel. If in doubt the 0.018 inch guidewire can be replaced in most cases by a 22G plastic cannula, which allows pressure to be measured and so can reliably exclude or confirm an intra-arterial cannula placement. Blood gas analysis is unreliable and should not be used for this. But even if the correct venous position is confirmed, damage to the vessel followed by massive and continuous bleeding after catheter placement can occur. The author remembers several such cases, especially following femoral venous cannulation.

In this case the **sympatholytic effects** of the caudal epidural block may have contributed to the timely recovery of the arterial circulation. This has anecdotally been reported after drug-induced vasospasm (Kessell & Barker 1996) and after ischaemia caused by a regional block (Kaplanian *et al.* 2007).

Summary and Recommendations

This case of blood vessel trauma shows that every effort is needed to cannulate the desired vessel in the first attempt; clinically this means by using ultrasound right from the beginning.

The most dangerous step (the 'real weapon' in the hands of the anaesthetist) during vascular catheterization is dilatation; before doing it one has to be 100% confident that the guidewire is lying in the desired venous vessel.

Using a blood pressure transducer will most reliably allow one to distinguish an arterial from a venous position. Blood gas analysis should not be used for this.

References

Bodenham, C.A., Babu, S., Bennett, J., *et al.* (2016). Association of Anaesthetists of Great Britain and Ireland: safe vascular access 2016. *Anaesthesia*, 71, 573–585.

Goobie, S.M., Cladis, F.P., Glover, C.D., *et al.* (2017). Safety of antifibrinolytics in cranial vault reconstructive surgery: a report from the pediatric craniofacial collaborative group. *Paediatr Anaesth*, 27, 271–281.

Kaplanian, S., Chambers, N.A., & Forsyth, I. (2007). Caudal anaesthesia as a treatment for penile ischaemia following circumcision. *Anaesthesia*, 62, 741–743.

Kessell, G. & Barker, I. (1996). Leg ischaemia in an infant following accidental intra-arterial administration of atracurium treated with caudal anaesthesia. *Anaesthesia*, 51, 1154–1156.

Lin, P.H., Dodson, T.F., Bush, R.L., *et al.* (2001). Surgical intervention for complications caused by femoral artery catheterization in pediatric patients. *J Vasc Surg*, 34, 1071–1078.

4.7

Malposition of the Catheter Tip

Case

A 3-year-old girl underwent laparoscopic appendectomy because of a perforated appendix with diffuse peritonitis. At the end of the case it was decided to insert a central venous catheter at the request of the surgeon, because of previous difficulties with venous access. A 4F double-lumen catheter was inserted at the first attempt under ultrasound guidance into the right internal jugular vein. Because the intervention took place out of hours, the decision was taken to forgo an immediate radiographic confirmation and to request a chest x-ray the next morning.

Two days later the nurses called the anaesthetist because blood could not be aspirated from the catheter for laboratory testing, and in addition there was a marked swelling of the right forearm (Fig. 4.7a). The girl, quite upset by the presence of medical staff, was transferred to the operating suite, accompanied by her parents. There she received intra-venous sedation with ketamine, and the ultrasound examination, now in a quiet child, showed a catheter malposition, with the catheter visible in the right subclavian vein. Because of the favourable clinical course, the central venous catheter was removed, and a peripheral line was inserted into the left cephalic vein at the forearm under ultrasound guidance. Obviously, by mistake, the requested radiographic check to exclude a catheter malposition had not taken place.

Discussion

This case of **catheter malposition** leading to partial thrombosis of the subclavian vein illustrates the importance of an established standard in dealing with these medical devices (Frykholm *et al.* 2014). In every single case, the correct position, in the superior (SVC) or inferior vena cava (IVC), has to be confirmed. This is traditionally done by radiography; an intravascular ECG is an alternative, but it depends on reaching an intracardiac position, from which the catheter is withdrawn until the typical high p-waves have consistently disappeared. But many paediatric catheter models are too short to guarantee this procedure in all patients. In addition, the 'busy ECG' at high heart rates may sometimes make the interpretation quite difficult. Ultrasound can be used – but whereas the IVC can be reliably visualized in neonates and small children, even by an inexperienced practitioner, the visibility of the SVC is limited by the presence of air-filled structures (Park *et al.* 2014). After subclavian puncture a catheter malposition occurs in up to 20%, but it is a relatively rare event when the right internal jugular vein is cannulated.

The **depth of insertion** can be reliably predicted for catheters inserted via the right internal jugular vein; body length divided by 10 gives a first guess, and then it can be estimated more precisely by directly measuring the distance from the point of insertion to the midpoint between the suprasternal notch and the intermammillary line (Jöhr 2013) or by more sophisticated formulas (Na *et al.* 2009). The goal is the placement of the catheter tip outside the heart in the SVC; this equates to a position near the carina on the chest x-ray. This calculation was done in our case; nevertheless, the malposition was still possible. For a femoral catheter an insertion depth of less than the distance from the puncture site to the xiphoid almost guarantees a position of the tip outside the heart. The distance from little finger to thumb of the practitioner's hand, 23 cm in the case of the author, can be used to estimate the maximally allowed depth of insertion. For all other insertion points the prediction of the correct insertion length is much less precise. An intracardiac position of the catheter tip carries the risk of an atrial wall perforation with a consequent cardiac tamponade (Orme *et al.* 2007). Numerous such cases have been reported in the literature, surprisingly often in the context of very thin peripherally inserted catheters in neonates (Warren *et al.* 2013); this makes toxic damage to the myocardium with subsequent necrosis more likely than an exclusively mechanical perforation. During his professional career the author was aware of three such cases, and was personally directly involved in one.

Malposition is of interest with **femoral** lines too (Lavandosky *et al.* 1996); in particular, catheters inserted from the left side can slip into paravertebral or even epidural veins, causing catastrophic neurological complications (Fig. 4.7b) (Zenker *et al.* 2000). To confirm

(a)

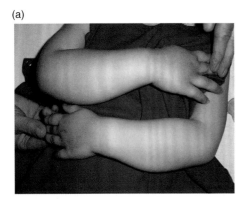

Figure 4.7a Malpositioned internal jugular catheter leading to a swelling of the right arm.

(b)

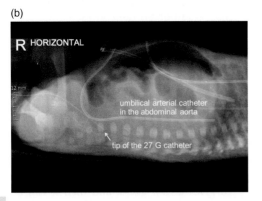

R HORIZONTAL

12 mm

umbilical arterial catheter in the abdominal aorta

tip of the 27 G catheter

Figure 4.7b This abdominal x-ray shows a malpositioned 27G catheter in a paravertebral vein; in addition, a pneumoperitoneum is clearly present.

the correct position an abdominal x-ray with a horizontal beam is recommended (Berger & Fontana 2016). The catheter should project anteriorly to the vertebral bodies, parallel to an umbilical artery catheter, if there is one in place. In addition, the author has witnessed the insertion of femoral catheters into the abdomen. In a trauma case, it is possible for blood to be aspirated from the abdomen too, and into the urinary bladder. Today, with ultrasound guidance, this will hopefully no longer occur. The optimal depth of insertion is not well defined for femoral lines, but the catheter tip is probably best positioned above the entry points of the renal veins (Frykholm *et al.* 2014).

Peripherally inserted central catheters have been very popular in neonatology for decades and are now increasingly used in older children too (Westergaard *et al.* 2013); the same considerations about correct position and depth of insertion apply.

Summary and Recommendations

This case of subclavian vein thrombosis illustrates that it is important to ensure a correct position of the central venous catheter tip in every single patient.

The tip of a central venous catheter has to be positioned in the vena cava outside the area covered by pericardium and outside the atrium.

After the insertion of a central venous catheter in the inferior half of the body, an abdominal x-ray with a horizontal beam technique will demonstrate that the catheter is probably in the IVC and for sure not in a paravertebral vein.

References

Berger, T.M. & Fontana, M. (2016). Horizontal beam technique to document position of percutaneously inserted central venous catheters. *Arch Dis Child Fetal Neonatal Ed*, 101, F89.

Frykholm, P., Pikwer, A., Hammarskjold, F., *et al.* (2014). Clinical guidelines on central venous catheterisation. Swedish Society of Anaesthesiology and Intensive Care Medicine. *Acta Anaesthesiol Scand*, 58, 508–524.

Jöhr, M. (2013). *Kinderanästhesie*, 8th edn. München, Elsevier.

Lavandosky, G., Gomez, R., & Montes, J. (1996). Potentially lethal misplacement of femoral central venous catheters. *Crit Care Med*, 24, 893–896.

Na, H.S., Kim, J.T., Kim, H.S., *et al.* (2009). Practical anatomic landmarks for determining the insertion depth of central venous catheter in paediatric patients. *Br J Anaesth*, 102, 820–823.

Orme, R.M., McSwiney, M.M., & Chamberlain-Webber, R.F. (2007). Fatal cardiac tamponade as a result of a peripherally inserted central venous catheter: a case report and review of the literature. *Br J Anaesth*, 99, 384–388.

Park, Y.H., Lee, J.H., Byon, H.J., *et al.* (2014). Transthoracic echocardiographic guidance for obtaining an optimal insertion length of internal jugular venous catheters in infants. *Paediatr Anaesth*, 24, 927–932.

Warren, M., Thompson, K.S., Popek, E.J., *et al.* (2013). Pericardial effusion and cardiac tamponade in neonates: sudden unexpected death associated with total parenteral nutrition via central venous catheterization. *Ann Clin Lab Sci*, 43, 163–171.

Westergaard, B., Classen, V., & Walther-Larsen, S. (2013). Peripherally inserted central catheters in infants and children: indications, techniques, complications and clinical recommendations. *Acta Anaesthesiol Scand*, 57, 278–287.

Zenker, M., Rupprecht, T., Hofbeck, M., *et al.* (2000). Paravertebral and intraspinal malposition of transfemoral central venous catheters in newborns. *J Pediatr*, 136, 837–840.

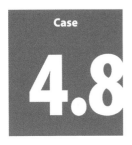

Anomalies of the Venous System

Case

Many years ago, a 3-month-old boy, 4.5 kg, was scheduled for major abdominal surgery. After induction of anaesthesia and endotracheal intubation the right internal jugular vein was punctured. Following guidewire insertion and dilatation a 4F double-lumen catheter was inserted.

During insertion of the guidewire an unfamiliar resistance was briefly felt, and at fluoroscopy the catheter was found deviating to the left. It was then further inserted until a position in the left-sided vena cava was obtained (Fig. 4.8).

Discussion

A **persistent left superior vena cava (PLSVC)** is the most common venous malformation, affecting 0.3–0.5% of the normal population; in patients with congenital heart disease the incidence is 3–5%, i.e. 10 times higher. Because the majority of central venous catheters are inserted via the right internal jugular or subclavian vein a PLSVC will remain undetected in many cases. The PLSVC runs anterior to the main pulmonary artery, angulates to the right and drains into a dilated coronary sinus. In the vast majority, over 90%, it is an additional vessel and a right vena cava exists too. Without cardiac surgery and venous cannulation it is mostly a trivial finding and does not interfere with normal life. In contrast to the right vena cava, the left vena cava is **angulated** and even may be **tortuous**. This makes the passage of guidewires more difficult and increases the risk of vessel perforation at dilatation or when stiff catheters are used (Balasubramanian *et al.* 2014). The insertion of pacemaker leads or pulmonary artery catheters is more demanding because of the additional angulation when entering the right atrium. Because of the angulated course the risk of thrombotic events may be increased in the presence of central venous catheters. Nevertheless, the PLSVC is a large central vessel and can be used in the same way as the right SVC for parenteral nutrition. The author remembers a neonate with PLSVC who needed parenteral nutrition over many weeks, and repeated central venous catheterization was performed using both sides; this was complicated by a thrombosis of the SVC on the left side, but not on the right side.

A left paratracheal position of the catheter on the x-ray is typical for a PLSVC; but an extravascular or intra-arterial position has to be taken into account too. However, in rare cases, a malposition in the **internal thoracic (mammary) vein** is possible (Kanbak *et al.* 2005). Compared to the vena cava this is a much smaller vessel, and the author remembers a case of early catheter dysfunction in a child with cancer in whom the misplacement into the right internal thoracic vein was not quickly recognized: a potentially

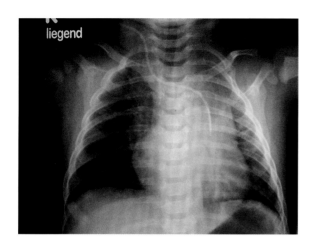

Figure 4.8 A persistent left superior vena cava (PLSVC) and a probably absent right superior vena cava.

life-threatening complication, as leakage of antineoplastic agents into the mediastinum would have been a disaster.

Inferior vena cava (IVC) anomalies, especially a double IVC, are present in 0.2–3% of the population (Bass *et al.* 2000). The right IVC usually follows the normal course, straight to the right atrium, whereas the left one angulates at the height of the entrance of the left renal vein and then joins the right venous system. Therefore, in the presence of a double IVC the right one should always be preferred for venous cannulation. In the presence of an azygos or hemiazygos continuation, the venous blood from the lower part of the body enters the right atrium from above. The majority of venous malformations remain unrecognized until intravascular catheters have to be placed (Yeung *et al.* 2016). Anomalies, especially agenesis of the IVC, may be connected with venous congestion and thrombosis (Milani *et al.* 2008).

In rare cases a PLSVC drains into the left atrium and causes a right-to-left shunt with central cyanosis. There is a huge variety of venous malformations, as illustrated by a vast number of case reports.

Summary and Recommendations

Anomalies of the venous system are relatively common; anatomy is not always normal, as we expect it, and a high index of suspicion is needed.

In the presence of a double vena cava (superior or inferior) the right system is usually less angulated and should be preferred for venous cannulation.

Even when cannulation is uneventful, the position of every central venous catheter has to be confirmed by an imaging technique.

References

Balasubramanian, S., Gupta, S., Nicholls, M., *et al.* (2014). Rare complication of a dialysis catheter insertion. *Clin Kidney J*, 7, 194–196.

Bass, J.E., Redwine, M.D., Kramer, L.A., *et al.* (2000). Spectrum of congenital anomalies of the inferior vena cava: cross-sectional imaging findings. *Radiographics*, 20, 639–652.

Kanbak, M., Karagoz, A.H., Oc, M., *et al.* (2005). Malposition of internal jugular catheter into internal mammarian vein in coronary artery bypass grafting. *Eur J Anaesthesiol*, 22, 399–400.

Milani, C., Constantinou, M., Berz, D., *et al.* (2008). Left sided inferior vena cava duplication and venous thromboembolism: case report and review of literature. *J Hematol Oncol*, 1, 24.

Yeung, N.P., Wong, C.C., Young, K., *et al.* (2016). Complication of venovenous extracorporeal membrane oxygenation cannulation: the significance of an inferior vena cava anomaly. *Clin Case Rep*, 4, 1132–1134.

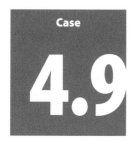

Air Embolism

Case

Many decades ago, a 3-year-old girl with hypoganglionosis, weighing 14 kg, was scheduled for abdominal revision surgery and removal of a leaking, but provisionally repaired Broviac catheter. A peripheral line and a new percutaneous central venous catheter were inserted on the opposite side, but the Broviac was still in use. Surgery involved releasing adhesions and caused continuous bleeding. After abdominal closure, surgery proceeded at the neck for the removal of the tunnelled Broviac catheter.

Up to this point the Broviac catheter was used for the application of blood products; one unit of packed red cells and a unit of fresh frozen plasma had been given. The intention was to empty the transfusion line, approximately 30 ml as the warming system was used, before removing it together with the Broviac catheter. Therefore the empty plasma bag was removed, and an already partly emptied bottle of Ringer's lactate was connected for flushing in the remaining plasma. At this time crystalloid solutions were still provided in glass bottles. But the drip was not running spontaneously, so the bottle was pressurized by pumping air into it. The head nurse admonished the anaesthetist to be careful, because pressurizing glass bottles was already considered a dangerous practice. When the catheter was due to be removed, the surgeon asked for the running infusion to be stopped, and then pulled out the catheter. Almost simultaneously, the pulse oximeter signal disappeared and bradycardia with wide QRS complexes developed. A dose of 50 μg adrenaline, approximately 3 μg/kg, was given from a prefilled syringe with minimal delay. Heart rate increased and within minutes the situation was stabilized. The clamped infusion tubing was found without fluid, but filled with air down to the Broviac catheter.

Discussion

It is very likely that **air embolism** caused the cardiovascular collapse. Happily the quantity of air was probably small and the outcome favourable, because the infusion tubing was attentively observed by the anaesthetist, who wanted to flush in only the remaining amount of plasma. Initially, because of the coincidence with the removal of the Broviac catheter, embolism of a fibrinous clot mobilized by the manipulations during catheter removal was considered as the most probable cause of the event; but then the air-filled tubing was noticed. The amount of air which is still safe is unknown; in a porcine model 2 ml/kg resulted in cardiac arrest (Richter *et al.* 2013); but in the presence of an open foramen ovale much smaller amounts could lead to a paradoxical embolism to the brain or the coronary arteries, with a catastrophic outcome.

Infusion therapy has the inherent risk of air embolism, as soon as a false manipulation is made. Air embolism can occur, even without the application of pressure or the presence of a pump; the volume of air that fills the intravenous tubing can be infused by gravity into the patient (Laskey *et al.* 2002). Simply forgetting to purge the air out of the tubing before connecting it to the patient can lead to fatal air embolism in an infant. The author is aware of such cases occurring in highly reputed institutions.

Whenever the venous system is open at a point above the level of the heart, air can potentially enter the circulation. Neurosurgical interventions in the **sitting position** inherently carry the risk of air embolism (Harrison *et al.* 2002). During craniosynostosis surgery the air enters via the open spongiosa, and detectable air embolism occurs in the majority of patients (Faberowski *et al.* 2000). Orthopaedic interventions, e.g. scoliosis surgery, where the cut spongious bone has contact with the atmosphere (Sutherland & Winter 1997), as well as hepatic resection with large open veins, are situations at risk. A rare but typical situation is gas embolism during the use of argon-enhanced coagulation systems (Veyckemans & Michel 1996). The insertion of large cannulas or sheaths, e.g. during cardiac catheterization or during the insertion of a central venous catheter, is always a risky situation.

During **laparoscopy** the elevated abdominal pressure allows the entrance of gas into the venous system as soon as a vessel wall is damaged. As the entrance of air into the venous system is much more dangerous than carbon dioxide, it is important to flush the insufflation tubing with carbon dioxide before connecting it with the trocar (Richter *et al.* 2013). In neonates the large still open umbilical vein at the site of trocar insertion carries additional risks, the passive entrance of air during the preparation phase (Lalwani & Aliason 2009) and the typical carbon dioxide embolism during the procedure (Olsen *et al.* 2013). Irrigating tissue cavities with a gas-forming solution such as **hydrogen peroxide** has also been reported to cause severe gas embolism (Gerrish 1985).

Pressurizing bags or glass bottles containing residual air has long been recognized as a dangerous manoeuvre (Adhikary & Massey 1998), and was already considered to fall short of **standard of care** at the time of the event. Nevertheless it was done; typically, the individual anaesthetist believes that in his own hands even a dubious procedure must be safe.

There is no doubt that the rapid administration of **adrenaline** had an impact on the benign course of the event. Adrenaline is only rarely used in paediatric anaesthesia; nevertheless it is of great benefit to have it drawn up in a syringe. The author had, since the early 1990s, a prefilled 10 ml syringe with adrenaline 100 μg/ml in the anaesthesia chart. Stability is maintained over several months and it allows almost immediate injection of the compound. The author believes that in hectic situations there is no time to draw up medications; a hypnotic, a relaxant, atropine and adrenaline should always be at hand and ready for injection.

Summary and Recommendations

Infusion therapy carries the inherent risk of venous air embolism, as soon as a wrong manipulation is made.

Prefilled syringes allow the rapid administration of life-saving medications such as adrenaline.

This case also shows that the individual anaesthetist proceeds with substandard care because he is convinced that in his own hands even a dubious procedure is safe.

References

Adhikary, G.S. & Massey, S.R. (1998). Massive air embolism: a case report. *J Clin Anesth*, 10, 70–72.

Faberowski, L.W., Black, S., & Mickle, J.P. (2000). Incidence of venous air embolism during craniectomy for craniosynostosis repair. *Anesthesiology*, 92, 20–23.

Gerrish, S.P. (1985). Gas embolism due to hydrogen peroxide. *Anaesthesia*, 40, 1244.

Harrison, E.A., Mackersie, A., McEwan, A., *et al.* (2002). The sitting position for neurosurgery in children: a review of 16 years' experience. *Br J Anaesth*, 88, 12–17.

Lalwani, K. & Aliason, I. (2009). Cardiac arrest in the neonate during laparoscopic surgery. *Anesth Analg*, 109, 760–762.

Laskey, A.L., Dyer, C., & Tobias, J.D. (2002). Venous air embolism during home infusion therapy. *Pediatrics*, 109, E15.

Olsen, M., Avery, N., Khurana, S., *et al.* (2013). Pneumoperitoneum for neonatal laparoscopy: how safe is it? *Paediatr Anaesth*, 23, 457–459.

Richter, S., Matthes, C., Ploenes, T., *et al.* (2013). Air in the insufflation tube may cause fatal embolizations in laparoscopic surgery: an animal study. *Surg Endosc*, 27, 1791–1797.

Sutherland, R.W. & Winter, R.J. (1997). Two cases of fatal air embolism in children undergoing scoliosis surgery. *Acta Anaesthesiol Scand*, 41, 1073–1076.

Veyckemans, F. & Michel, I. (1996). Venous gas embolism from an argon coagulator. *Anesthesiology*, 85, 443–444.

Case

A long time ago, an 11-year-old girl with slipped capital femoral epiphysis (SCFE) underwent reduction and fixation of the right femoral head under general endotracheal anaesthesia; in addition a femoral nerve block had been performed for postoperative analgesia. The contralateral side was fixed with pins prophylactically. On the second postoperative day a marked swelling of both legs was seen.

Further investigation led to the diagnosis of a thrombosis predominantly of the right femoral vein extending to the inferior vena cava. Intravenous heparin was given and the advice of a specialized vascular surgeon was sought; in view of the extensive spread of the thrombus he recommended a surgical thrombectomy, which was subsequently performed under general endotracheal anaesthesia. Surprisingly, the further investigations showed no signs of pathology in the coagulation system, especially no inherited thrombophilia.

Discussion

This case illustrates that manifest postoperative deep **venous thrombosis** is a rare (Georgopoulos *et al.* 2016), but not absent phenomenon. Routine prophylactic medication for all paediatric patients is not an established practice; however, it may be wise to provide prophylaxis against venous thromboembolism, similarly to adult practice, to some patients beyond a certain age and at higher risk. In the author's institution this age limit for the administration of prophylactic low-molecular-weight heparin in the context of surgery was set arbitrarily at 13 years for girls and 15 years for boys. This could be considered overzealous, because overall the risk seems to be low even after prolonged surgery (Kaabachi *et al.* 2010). However, the paediatric spectrum also includes patients who are definitely at a higher risk, e.g. the adipose girl taking contraceptive medication. Therefore the topic has to be in the focus of the paediatric anaesthetist, and a clear institutional policy is mandatory.

After the **neonatal period** and before puberty, venous thrombosis is a rare event in paediatric patients (Tuckuviene *et al.* 2011). During infancy the incidence is higher in boys than in girls, but during adolescence the opposite is the case. A **central venous catheter** is the single most predictive factor for venous thromboembolism in children (Kim & Sabharwal 2014). In neonates an extremely high incidence of venous thromboembolism is observed (Latham & Thompson 2014) and over 90% of the thrombotic events are catheter-related (Chalmers 2006).

There is no unequivocal proof of the effectiveness of low-molecular-weight heparin or the use of heparin-bonded catheters for the prevention of catheter-related thrombosis

(Brandao *et al.* 2014). In neonates, some institutions infuse 0.5 U/kg/h of heparin to keep the central venous catheter open. In the presence of a confirmed catheter-related thrombosis it is recommended to remove the catheter after 3–5 days of therapeutic anticoagulation (Monagle *et al.* 2012); if during the follow-up an extension of the thrombus is observed, anticoagulation for 6 weeks to 3 months has to be considered. The author has to admit that over the last 10 years, with the ubiquitous use of ultrasound, he has often seen a small thrombus formation when there is a catheter in place and has often ignored it as a 'normal' benign phenomenon (Fig. 4.10a).

The extensive experience with dilatation and revascularization of partially occluded vessels for renal replacement therapy indicates that it is probably safe to manipulate and to puncture these partially occluded vessels for the insertion of a new catheter; the risk of dislodging a thrombus seems to be low. These small local phenomena are different to the thrombotic occlusion of the superior or inferior vena cava, a potentially life-threatening event. A congestion of the distant part of the body and a collateral circulation is often visible (Fig. 4.10b). The author has seen several such cases, all in neonates; when a percutaneously inserted 4F double-lumen catheter was used, typically a leakage at the insertion site occurred, and the infused fluid oozed back along a fibrinous sheet covering the catheter.

Inherited thrombophilia is quite common, but it rarely leads to unprovoked thrombosis in neonates and children (van Ommen & Nowak-Gottl 2017). Therefore, before puberty, and in contrast to adults, prophylactic medication is usually not given for minor low-risk surgery. The most common defect is factor V Leiden mutation, with an incidence

(a)

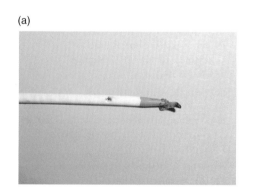

Figure 4.10a This thrombus obstructing the distal orifice of a central venous catheter was an incidental finding.

(b)

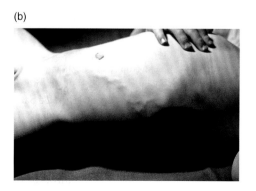

Figure 4.10b This boy with an obvious bypassing venous circulation presented for further investigations a few years after long-term parenteral nutrition during the neonatal period.

of 1–9% within Europe, followed by factor II mutation with 2%. In unclear situations the advice of a specialist must be sought. Similarly to adults, **malignancy** is a risk factor for thrombotic events in children. Asparaginase, which is used in the treatment of acute lymphoblastic leukaemia, induces an antithrombin deficiency (Tuckuviene *et al.* 2016).

Some types of **surgery** typically predispose to localized thrombotic events, e.g. portal vein thrombosis connected with laparoscopic splenectomy or interventions close to the porta hepatis.

Summary and Recommendations

Thromboembolic events are rare after routine paediatric surgery. However, they do occur, and prophylactic medication is worthwhile in adolescence and in situations with a specific risk.

Neonates are at a high risk for thrombotic events, especially in connection with central venous catheters. Thinner catheters may be preferable.

Inherited thrombophilia is not a major risk during routine paediatric surgery.

References

Brandao, L.R., Shah, N., & Shah, P.S. (2014). Low molecular weight heparin for prevention of central venous catheterization-related thrombosis in children. *Cochrane Database Syst Rev*, (3), CD005982.

Chalmers, E.A. (2006). Epidemiology of venous thromboembolism in neonates and children. *Thromb Res*, 118, 3–12.

Georgopoulos, G., Hotchkiss, M.S., McNair, B., *et al.* (2016). Incidence of deep vein thrombosis and pulmonary embolism in the elective pediatric orthopaedic patient. *J Pediatr Orthop*, 36, 101–109.

Kaabachi, O., Alkaissi, A., Koubaa, W., *et al.* (2010). Screening for deep venous thrombosis after idiopathic scoliosis surgery in children: a pilot study. *Paediatr Anaesth*, 20, 144–149.

Kim, S.J. & Sabharwal, S. (2014). Risk factors for venous thromboembolism in hospitalized children and adolescents: a systemic review and pooled analysis. *J Pediatr Orthop B*, 23, 389–393.

Latham, G.J. & Thompson, D.R. (2014). Thrombotic complications in children from short-term percutaneous central venous catheters: what can we do? *Paediatr Anaesth*, 24, 902–911.

Monagle, P., Chan, A.K.C., Goldenberg, N.A., *et al.* (2012). Antithrombotic therapy in neonates and children: antithrombotic therapy and prevention of thrombosis, 9th ed: American College of Chest Physicians Evidence-Based Clinical Practice Guidelines. *Chest*, 141 (2 Suppl.), e737S–e801S.

Tuckuviene, R., Christensen, A.L., Helgestad, J., *et al.* (2011). Pediatric venous and arterial noncerebral thromboembolism in Denmark: a nationwide population-based study. *J Pediatr*, 159, 663–669.

Tuckuviene, R., Ranta, S., Albertsen, B.K., *et al.* (2016). Prospective study of thromboembolism in 1038 children with acute lymphoblastic leukemia: a Nordic Society of Pediatric Hematology and Oncology (NOPHO) study. *J Thromb Haemost*, 14, 485–494.

van Ommen, C.H. & Nowak-Gottl, U. (2017). Inherited thrombophilia in pediatric venous thromboembolic disease: why and who to test. *Front Pediatr*, 5, 50.

Ischaemic Fingers

Case

Many years ago, a term neonate, weighing 2.5 kg, was scheduled for a laparotomy because of intestinal obstruction. After induction with thiopental and pancuronium the trachea was intubated with a size 3.0 uncuffed endotracheal tube, and anaesthesia was maintained with fentanyl and sevoflurane.

The arterial cannulation was rather time-consuming but finally successful using a 22G steel needle and a 2F catheter inserted by the Seldinger technique. The catheter was connected to the extension tubing and continuously flushed with normal saline with 2 U/ml heparin at a rate of 2 ml/h. The hand was cleaned and in accordance with local protocol fixed on a splint. At that moment white fingers were noticed (Fig. 4.11). Repeated flushing did not alter the situation, and, in addition, the arterial curve showed a damped tracing. It was only about half an hour later, following skin incision, when mean arterial pressure was well above 40 mmHg, that suddenly a normal arterial tracing was visible, and all the fingers now turned pink.

Discussion

This case illustrates the concerns of the paediatric anaesthetist when dealing with **arterial catheters** in neonates and small infants. It focuses attention on several educational points.

First, the **technique of insertion** has changed over time; in the early 1980s the author occasionally had recourse to a surgical cut-down when the palpation method failed, then the period of transillumination came, and today the ultrasound-based approach has become his preferred method in all patients (Anantasit *et al.* 2017). A 24G plastic cannula, e.g. Insyte or Vasofix, may be a good choice, because it causes minimal trauma and usually no relevant haematoma when the artery is punctured repeatedly. In neonates low blood pressure and the high haematocrit often create additional difficulties, because the backflow is often hesitant. Although the author preferred the Seldinger technique he had the impression that, in the short term, directly introduced catheters performed better than those inserted over a guidewire.

Second, in neonates the preferred **site of insertion** is the right radial artery, because it allows a preductal sampling of blood gases; however, the ulnar vessel is often bigger and easier to cannulate. Because of the risk of ischaemia, it is clearly unwise to proceed to the ulnar artery when the radial artery has already been punctured but threading the catheter was unsuccessful. The axillary artery is a large vessel, relatively easy to cannulate, and when the puncture is made high up in the axilla, there is a large collateral network (Piotrowski & Kawczynski 1995); in the classic Blalock–Taussig procedure the subclavian artery was even

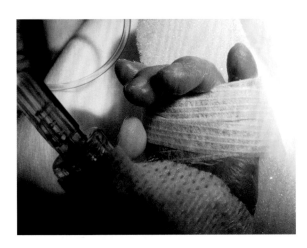

Figure 4.11 Ischaemic fingertips after the insertion of a radial artery catheter (from Jöhr, M. (2017). Complications in paediatric anaesthesia. *Anästh Intensivmed*, 58, 259–266, with permission).

cut and ligated. The only disadvantage is its vicinity to the cerebral circulation. The author remembers only one child who developed a pulseless arm after several days on the ICU with a catheter in the axillary artery. The catheter was withdrawn and the circulation gradually returned. The brachial artery has been used successfully by some authorities (Schindler *et al.* 2005). In preterm and term neonates cannulation of the femoral artery probably carries a risk of leg ischaemia (Venkataraman *et al.* 1997); it was, because of negative experience by the author, always the last choice in this age group. The posterior tibial artery is widely used in neonatology. The author used it only when other access sites had failed, because finger ischaemia is not common in a geriatric population, but necrotic toes are – and it may be that even a small scar in the intima of a foot vessel will have negative consequences many decades later.

Third, in the presented case finger ischaemia was probably caused by the **embolization** of small bubbles of air. This was supported by the transient nature of the phenomenon. Continuous flushing with a heparin-containing solution is used by most practitioners for paediatric patients. Flushing by injecting a bolus is sometimes done, but it is potentially hazardous because the solution and the potentially included thrombotic material can retrogradely reach the central circulation. Even in adults a volume of only 3 ml seems to be sufficient (Lowenstein *et al.* 1971), and it will be much less in neonates and infants. Those patients with axillary or, worse, temporal artery catheters are especially at risk. Temporal artery catheters were banned from clinical practice a long time ago after reports of brain infarcts (Prian *et al.* 1978, Simmons *et al.* 1978). With axillary catheters the distance is greater when the left side is cannulated.

Persistent **ischaemia** with necrosis has been reported and is a continuous threat. In case of disturbed perfusion it is always wise to check for adequate blood pressure. As in the presented case, simply increasing blood pressure well above 40 mmHg in neonates will completely restore perfusion. The probable result of this increase in pressure was to eliminate the spasm and to flush away the minimal thrombotic material. In neonates and small infants, areas of skin necrosis at the site overlying the catheter tip are typically seen in up to 10% of cases. In the absence of sepsis and shock, or damage to multiple vessels, a limb-threatening ischaemia rarely occurs. The author remembers a 2-year-old boy who survived a toxic shock syndrome after weeks of ICU treatment but lost tissue on all four extremities;

the necrosis was far more severe on the side of the arterial line. It is usually sufficient to remove the catheter and to ensure that there is sufficient perfusion pressure. Other potential treatment modalities are heparin, fibrinolysis and vasodilatation by a sympathetic block.

Summary and Recommendations

This case of transient fingertip ischaemia emphasizes the importance of avoiding even the smallest air bubbles in the tubing.

Flushing should be performed with the smallest effective volume, approximately 0.5 ml in a neonate, in order to avoid embolization into the central, especially the cerebral, circulation.

References

Anantasit, N., Cheeptinnakorntaworn, P., Khositseth, A., *et al.* (2017). Ultrasound versus traditional palpation to guide radial artery cannulation in critically ill children: a randomized trial. *J Ultrasound Med*, 36, 2495–2501.

Lowenstein, E., Little, J.W. III, & Lo, H.H. (1971). Prevention of cerebral embolization from flushing radial-artery cannulas. *N Engl J Med*, 285, 1414–1415.

Piotrowski, A. & Kawczynski, P. (1995). Cannulation of the axillary artery in critically ill newborn infants. *Eur J Pediatr*, 154, 57–59.

Prian, G.W., Wright, G.B., Rumack, C.M., *et al.* (1978). Apparent cerebral embolization after temporal artery catheterization. *J Pediatr*, 93, 115–118.

Schindler, E., Kowald, B., Suess, H., *et al.* (2005). Catheterization of the radial or brachial artery in neonates and infants. *Paediatr Anaesth*, 15, 677–682.

Simmons, M.A., Levine, R.L., Lubchenco, L.O., *et al.* (1978). Warning: serious sequelae of temporal artery catheterization. *J Pediatr*, 92, 284.

Venkataraman, S.T., Thompson, A.E., & Orr, R.A. (1997). Femoral vascular catheterization in critically ill infants and children. *Clin Pediatr (Phila)*, 36, 311–319.

5 Regional Anaesthesia

Wrong-Site Block

Case

Decades ago, an 11-year-old girl with a history of previous bilateral clubfoot surgery as an infant was scheduled for unilateral corrective osteotomy at the foot level. After an inhalational induction a size 3 classic type laryngeal mask airway (LMA) was inserted and a proximal sciatic nerve block using the lateral approach was performed in the spontaneously breathing child. An advanced skilled resident was guided by the senior anaesthetist. The right foot was taped in a slight inwards rotation in order to elevate the greater trochanter, the position of which was then marked on the skin, and after extensive skin disinfection a 10 cm long isolated nerve stimulator needle was advanced below the greater trochanter in parallel to the surface of the table until the typical twitches appeared. The current was then turned down and 20 ml of bupivacaine 0.25% was injected at a site where, with 0.3 mA using an impulse width of 1 ms, twitches were no longer visible. Photos were taken during the procedure for future teaching purposes, including one showing the happy and proud resident. The right hip area was cleaned, the patient transferred from the induction room to theatre, and there the resident took further care of the patient.

Ten minutes later, he stuck his head out of the door of the theatre and said 'everything is fine, but surgery is intended to be on the left side.' Indeed, on the surgical list, a left-sided osteotomy was scheduled, as had been written on the anaesthetic chart at the time of the pre-anaesthetic visit. While the girl was still in theatre, the parents were seen on the ward by the anaesthetist and informed face to face about the mishap. At the end of the case a left-sided sciatic nerve block was performed, which provided long-lasting postoperative analgesia.

Discussion

This case shows that **wrong-site blocks** can occur, even in the context of scheduled routine surgery. A wrong-site block is a 'never event' and one of the most preventable medical errors. It is always a matter of negligence at some point. Nevertheless, the author was directly involved in this case and is aware of two other cases. In the literature an **incidence** in the range of 1–4 per 10000 blocks has been reported (Hudson *et al.* 2015, Sites *et al.* 2014), predominantly involving femoral nerve blocks, and the topic has been the focus of review articles (Barrington *et al.* 2015). Naturally the risk of wrong-site blocks exists for pain blocks too (Cohen *et al.* 2010).

The most relevant **risk factors** are distraction, fatigue and unusual production pressure. In addition, as in this case, the blocked wrong extremity often shows some abnormalities, e.g. a cast, a scar or a malformation. It is of paramount importance not to perform the block on the **apparently affected** extremity, but to assure oneself that this existing pathology is indeed the target of surgery. In addition, every **change in position**, e.g. from supine to lateral or from lateral to prone, increases the risk of a right–left error.

For **prevention** it is important to check all documentation and to verify the site marking. The WHO surgical checklist has undoubtedly brought more stability to the perioperative process (Haynes *et al.* 2009). Recently a specific checklist for performing regional blocks has been proposed (Mulroy *et al.* 2014). The author uses a very simple spoken checklist before inducing general anaesthesia (cf. Case 2.1) and since this case a brief pause before inserting the block needle in order to check the side. Marking the surgical site was not yet standard practice in those days; a visible mark on the left foot would have undoubtedly prevented proceeding with a sciatic nerve block on the right side. In this case there was no hectic atmosphere and no distraction; the teaching senior anaesthetist saw the right foot with its abnormal appearance, and was so convinced that it must be the right side that the trainee didn't question this.

The '**stop before you block**' initiative recommends a pre-procedure pause to confirm the correct side for the regional anaesthetic block. The success of such an initiative relies on repeated education and necessitates a change in culture; especially in emergency cases and in out-of-theatre procedures, the site check often gets forgotten (Slocombe & Pattullo 2016). Unhappily, despite special efforts, the incidence of wrong-site blocks seems to have remained stable over the years (Pandit *et al.* 2017). To increase adherence to the 'stop before you block' checklist, a suggestion has been made to mark the block site and to use special stickers on the syringe (Chikkabbaiah *et al.* 2015). And recently the performance of a 'mock block', touching the skin with an empty syringe and so challenging the awake patient to confirm the side, has been suggested (Pandit *et al.* 2017).

Unfortunately, humans are only reliably protected against mistakes which they have already made themselves, and through which they have acquired their own hurtful experience. The author, as well as the former resident, now head of a department, still remember this story well, a little ashamed but with the passage of time also with a big smile. It is very likely that these two anaesthetists are well protected against performing wrong-site blocks in the future.

Summary and Recommendations

Wrong-site block is an ever-present threat, and every effort should be made to avoid it.

A visibly affected extremity may not be the target of surgery; one should never proceed without checking all the documentation and the marking on the skin.

A short break before inserting the needle and checking the side and the indication ('stop before you block') is strongly recommended.

References

Barrington, M.J., Uda, Y., Pattullo, S.J., *et al.* (2015). Wrong-site regional anesthesia: review and recommendations for prevention? *Curr Opin Anaesthesiol*, 28, 670–684.

Chikkabbaiah, V., French, J., Townsley, P., *et al.* (2015). Further reducing the risk of wrong site block. *Anaesthesia*, 70, 1453.

Cohen, S.P., Hayek, S.M., Datta, S., *et al.* (2010). Incidence and root cause analysis of wrong-site pain management procedures: a multicenter study. *Anesthesiology*, 112, 711–718.

Haynes, A.B., Weiser, T.G., Berry, W.R., *et al.* (2009). A surgical safety checklist to reduce morbidity and mortality in a global population. *N Engl J Med*, 360, 491–499.

Hudson, M.E., Chelly, J.E., & Lichter, J.R. (2015). Wrong-site nerve blocks: 10 yr experience in a large multihospital health-care system. *Br J Anaesth*, 114, 818–824.

Mulroy, M.F., Weller, R.S., & Liguori, G.A. (2014). A checklist for performing regional nerve blocks. *Reg Anesth Pain Med*, 39, 195–199.

Pandit, J.J., Matthews, J., & Pandit, M. (2017). 'Mock before you block': an in-built action-check to prevent wrong-side anaesthetic nerve blocks. *Anaesthesia*, 72, 150–155.

Sites, B.D., Barrington, M.J., & Davis, M. (2014). Using an international clinical registry of regional anesthesia to identify targets for quality improvement. *Reg Anesth Pain Med*, 39, 487–495.

Slocombe, P. & Pattullo, S. (2016). A site check prior to regional anaesthesia to prevent wrong-sided blocks. *Anaesth Intensive Care*, 44, 513–516.

Case

A long time ago, a 14-year-old boy with Duchenne muscular dystrophy, weighing 28 kg, was scheduled for bilateral tenotomy of the Achilles tendon and the tendon of the tibialis posterior muscle (needing an incision close to the medial malleolus). He had lost ambulation at the age of 8 and was on non-invasive BIPAP ventilation during the night since the age of 12. He had been seen in the outpatient clinic several weeks earlier, and a spinal anaesthetic was planned.

On the day of surgery, remifentanil 0.1 µg/kg/min was administered and he was positioned in the left lateral position for performing the spinal block; now an impressive scar was visible from the thoracic level down to the sacrum – obviously following scoliosis surgery and spondylodesis around a year ago. The anaesthetist requested to see the x-ray of the spine, but it was unavailable because this procedure had been carried out in another hospital. Several attempts with a 27G Whitacre needle using the paramedian approach at the L5/S1 level failed, as did an attempt to perform a caudal block. While the anaesthetist persevered with the regional block attempts, nitrous oxide, repeated boluses of propofol and finally sevoflurane were administered because the patient was obviously suffering pain. Finally a laryngeal mask airway (LMA) was placed and anaesthesia was maintained with sevoflurane up to 0.5 MAC and remifentanil. Bilateral ultrasound-guided distal sciatic nerve block was performed with 15 ml bupivacaine 0.25% on each side. Muscle twitches could not be elicited.

At the end of surgery, with the intention of speeding up the surgical list, the surgeon requested to wake up the patient, to send him to the ICU and to apply the reductive cast later in the afternoon, because he considered this be a non-painful procedure. However, redressing the foot was painful, and so the cast had to be applied later, again under general anaesthesia, now using a total intravenous technique.

Discussion

This case emphasizes several educational points:

First, the chosen **regional technique** should reliably cover the whole field of surgery. The tendon of the tibialis posterior muscle inserts at the navicular bone of the foot, the tendon is running behind the tibia, and the skin incision for tenotomy is made close to the medial malleolus. Until recently it was the predominant belief that the very variable saphenous nerve exclusively covered the skin, and that the deeper structures were all innervated by the sciatic nerve. However, recent evidence shows that the saphenous nerve also has branches to the periosteum of the tibia and the medial talocrural capsule (Eglitis *et al.* 2016). Therefore, to cover the whole foot, e.g. for hallux valgus surgery, fixation of an os tibiale externum, or as in this case a tibialis posterior tenotomy, both a sciatic nerve block and a saphenous nerve block, or more proximally a femoral nerve block, have to be applied (Fig. 5.2a). In this case, the non-blocked saphenous nerve most likely explains the pain felt during the trial to apply the cast with the patient awake.

Second, **spinal anaesthesia** would have been an excellent choice in this high-risk patient with muscular dystrophy dependent on non-invasive ventilation during the night. Neuraxial anaesthesia can be successfully performed in patients with previous scoliosis surgery, although it is more demanding and has a higher failure rate (Ko & Leffert 2009). The responsible senior paediatric anaesthetist had successfully managed several such cases before. But in most of the reported cases in the literature scoliosis surgery did not involve the lower lumbar segments and the main difficulty was mastering the torsion of the spine. Choosing the L5/S1 interspace, the so-called Taylor's approach, is usually successful, because at this level the distortion of the spine is still minimal. But in the case presented here the scar went down to the sacrum and information about the exact extent of the previous surgery was unobtainable. Nevertheless, the preoperative evaluation had been done some time in advance and it would have been part of good practice to request the spine x-rays from the other hospital, to study them, and to choose then the best interspace or to abandon the plan for spinal anaesthesia. **Caudal anaesthesia** can be done in adolescents too (Keplinger *et al.* 2016), and is always an option after spine surgery because this area usually remains untouched by surgery (Fig. 5.2b). As only the segments distal to L4 would need to be blocked, moderate volumes of local anaesthetics would have been sufficient. Unfortunately the anaesthetist failed to identify the sacral epidural space and abandoned the technique mainly because it caused discomfort to the patient; in addition, at that date, experience with ultrasound for neuraxial anaesthesia was still limited.

Third, patients with **Duchenne muscular dystrophy** present a high risk for anaesthesia, even when surgery is only minor. The disease is an X-linked recessively

(a)

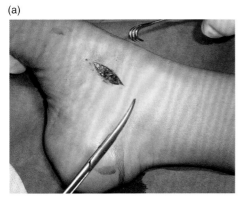

(b)

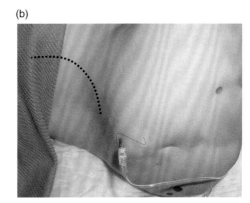

Figure 5.2a A sciatic and a saphenous nerve block are both needed to guarantee a completely pain-free child after surgery involving the medial aspects of the ankle.

Figure 5.2b Caudal block can be successfully performed in most children with severe scoliosis. This photo shows another child; in the presented patient, unfortunately, this was not the case.

inherited dystrophinopathy with an incidence of 1:4000. It is the most common myopathy. Dystrophin is a large protein responsible for the integrity of the sarcolemma (Segura *et al.* 2013). It is completely absent in Duchenne muscular dystrophy and it has an abnormal structure in Becker muscular dystrophy, which has a slower progression. Patients with Duchenne muscular dystrophy not only have progressive muscular weakness, which is usually apparent by 2 or 3 years of age, but also cardiomyopathy. Cardiac involvement can also be present in female carriers of the afflicted gene. Life expectancy has dramatically changed over the last few decades: today, with home ventilation, survival into the forties is no longer unusual (Kieny *et al.* 2013). Therefore every anaesthetist now has the potential to be exposed to such a patient.

The defect in the dystrophin–glycoprotein complex causes chronic instability of the cell membrane which is further enhanced by the administration of **succinylcholine** and to a lesser extent by inhalational agents (Schieren *et al.* 2017). The administration of succinylcholine leads to rhabdomyolysis and massive, often lethal hyperkalaemia; this is a particularly serious problem in the early stages of the disease, when the diagnosis is often not yet known and the absolute amount of muscle is still significant. The potential of having patients with undiagnosed muscular dystrophy was the main driver in banning succinylcholine from elective paediatric anaesthesia. Succinylcholine is definitively contraindicated in patients with Duchenne disease. These children do not have an increased risk of **malignant hyperthermia** susceptibility compared to the normal population (Gurnaney *et al.* 2009), but occasional cases of **rhabdomyolysis** following sevoflurane, without the other typical features of malignant hyperthermia, have been reported (Simpson & Van 2013). There is some consensus that for an elective case total intravenous anaesthesia is the preferred choice; but, because difficulties with venous access are very common in this group of patients, the majority of paediatric anaesthetists would take the advantages of an inhalational induction (Brandom & Veyckemans 2013). It is noteworthy that the incidence of anaesthesia-induced rhabdomyolysis is much lower than the incidence of Duchenne disease, and in a large series of children presenting for muscle biopsies inhalational agents have been used uneventfully, although some of them later proved to have Duchenne muscular dystrophy (Flick *et al.* 2007).

In the presented case, the option to administer sevoflurane for a short time was not taken 'voluntarily', as a first choice, but because the situation evolved from slight sedation to general anaesthesia in a suffering patient, and sevoflurane was ready at hand. For the second anaesthetic, the classic approach of a total intravenous anaesthesia was chosen.

Summary and Recommendations

This case shows that for covering all deep structures of the foot not only a sciatic but also a saphenous nerve block is needed.

A complete preoperative workup including a clinical examination and looking at the radiological findings would have prevented the unsuccessful attempts to perform a spinal block.

Patients with Duchenne muscular dystrophy are at high risk for perioperative complications. Whereas succinylcholine must not be given, inhalational agents may be used if clearly beneficial, e.g. in case of difficult vascular access.

References

Brandom, B.W. & Veyckemans, F. (2013). Neuromuscular diseases in children: a practical approach. *Paediatr Anaesth*, 23, 765–769.

Eglitis, N., Horn, J.L., Benninger, B., *et al.* (2016). The importance of the saphenous nerve in ankle surgery. *Anesth Analg*, 122, 1704–1706.

Flick, R.P., Gleich, S.J., Herr, M.M., *et al.* (2007). The risk of malignant hyperthermia in children undergoing muscle biopsy for suspected neuromuscular disorder. *Paediatr Anaesth*, 17, 22–27.

Gurnaney, H., Brown, A., & Litman, R.S. (2009). Malignant hyperthermia and muscular dystrophies. *Anesth Analg*, 109, 1043–1048.

Keplinger, M., Marhofer, P., Klug, W., *et al.* (2016). Feasibility and pharmacokinetics of caudal blockade in children and adolescents with 30–50 kg of body weight. *Paediatr Anaesth*, 26, 1053–1059.

Kieny, P., Chollet, S., Delalande, P., *et al.* (2013). Evolution of life expectancy of patients with Duchenne muscular dystrophy at AFM Yolaine de Kepper centre between 1981 and 2011. *Ann Phys Rehabil Med*, 56, 443–454.

Ko, J.Y. & Leffert, L.R. (2009). Clinical implications of neuraxial anesthesia in the parturient with scoliosis. *Anesth Analg*, 109, 1930–1934.

Schieren, M., Defosse, J., Böhmer, A., *et al.* (2017). Anaesthetic management of patients with myopathies. *Eur J Anaesthesiol*, 34, 641–649.

Segura, L.G., Lorenz, J.D., Weingarten, T.N., *et al.* (2013). Anesthesia and Duchenne or Becker muscular dystrophy: review of 117 anesthetic exposures. *Paediatr Anaesth*, 23, 855–864.

Simpson, R.S. & Van, K. (2013). Fatal rhabdomyolysis following volatile induction in a six-year-old boy with Duchenne muscular dystrophy. *Anaesth Intensive Care*, 41, 805–807.

Case
5.3
Undesirable Block Extension

Case

Decades ago, a 10-year-old girl, weighing 33 kg, was scheduled for bat ear surgery. After an inhalational induction and the administration of atracurium the airway was secured with a size 6.5 preformed endotracheal tube. Anaesthesia was maintained with nitrous oxide and halothane. The area of the retroauricular skin incision was infiltrated with 8 ml bupivacaine 0.25% with adrenaline 7.5 μg/ml on each side in order to provide a bloodless field and postoperative analgesia. The perioperative course was uneventful; the child was extubated and transferred to the surgical ward.

About 1 hour later, on the postoperative visit, the child was found with a complete right-sided facial nerve palsy with the inability to close the right eye. These findings worried the nursing staff; surprisingly, the child and her parents accepted this as a normal phenomenon after bat ear surgery. Because the anaesthetic course was completely uneventful and no other neurologic deficit was present, a causal relation with the bupivacaine infiltration was thought to be the most likely explanation, and the decision was taken only to observe the patient; indeed, after 6 more hours the facial weakness had disappeared.

Discussion

This case of **facial nerve palsy**, which has been previously reported in part elsewhere (Jöhr & Sossai 1996), illustrates that any local infiltration extending to the mastoid carries the risk of a facial nerve block. This can be frightening for the parents and especially puts the child at risk of corneal erosions, as reflexes such as protective lid closure are impeded. It is often wise to forgo wound infiltration around the face, especially in the mastoid area or lateral to the eye, when the local anaesthetic is exclusively given for postoperative analgesia and the child has a general anaesthetic anyway. Facial nerve palsy has also been reported after infiltration at the neck, e.g. for carotid artery surgery (Hayek *et al.* 2003).

Accidentally blocking the **vagus nerve** leads to vocal cord paralysis, with transient hoarseness, or in case of bilateral block to respiratory insufficiency. This can happen high up in the neck with infiltration of the tonsillar bed for postoperative analgesia (Weksler *et al.* 2001) or during infiltration in the vicinity of the carotid sheath (Thermann *et al.* 2007). Spread to the **phrenic nerve** is a typical side effect of interscalene brachial plexus block, but it can be accidentally blocked by any undirected deep infiltration at the neck (Schiessler *et al.* 1989).

A **Horner syndrome** with ptosis, miosis, enophthalmos and ipsilateral hyperaemia occurs through a high thoracic sympathetic blockade, e.g. by epidural anaesthesia, or a direct spread to the stellate ganglion, e.g. following an interscalene plexus block. It causes per se no major problems except the unexpected appearance; but miosis or more important anisocoric pupils can create diagnostic uncertainty and trigger unnecessary investigations. Therefore, the anaesthetist in charge has the responsibility to inform parents and medical staff about the benign nature of this phenomenon. Because of the proximity of the anatomic structures and the loose connective tissue enhancing the spread of injected solutions, a Horner syndrome is quite common in paediatric patients. The author has seen a Horner syndrome after an ultrasound-guided infraclavicular block in a school-aged child.

A Horner syndrome is often seen in the context of **epidural blockade**, with a vast number of reports in the literature (Aronson *et al.* 2000). The main issue is that a bilateral Horner syndrome is almost impossible to diagnose, because anisocoric pupils, the predominant diagnostic criterion, are not present; therefore Horner syndrome is only realized in the context of an asymmetrical spread of the epidural block. There are reports of a late appearance of Horner syndrome during a continuous epidural infusion of local anaesthetics, often after many hours or even days (Courtman & Carr 2000). However, such reports probably do not reflect a sudden higher, and therefore worrying, spread of the epidural blockade on the affected side; rather, the blocked area during an epidural infusion naturally regresses over time and suddenly Horner syndrome disappears on one side because of an asymmetrical regression of the blockade. In the author's practice, the presence of a Horner syndrome during well-functioning epidural analgesia was rarely a reason to reduce the infusion rate as long as motor impairment of the upper extremity was absent. The author has recently seen a Horner syndrome in an 8-month-old infant, weighing 6 kg, following a second caudal block with 1 ml/kg of ropivacaine 0.2% performed after urologic surgery with a delay of more than 3 hours after the first block (Fig. 5.3); and as usual, at first glance, unexplained anisocoric pupils at emergence frightened the anaesthetist.

In contrast to the transient nature of a Horner syndrome after local anaesthetics, stretching neural structures or a direct needle trauma can cause long-lasting symptoms. The author remembers, decades ago, a permanent Horner syndrome, or at least one that persisted over several months, after multiple trials to insert an internal jugular line. It has to be noted that moderate **anisocoria** is a physiological phenomenon; a pupil difference of 1 mm or more occurs naturally in 2.5% of children (Silbert *et al.* 2013). The author remembers several children who developed transient anisocoria during general anaesthesia

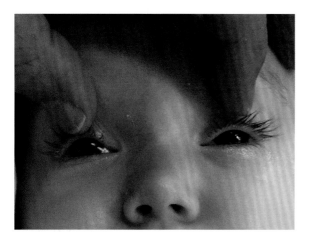

Figure 5.3 A transient Horner syndrome in an infant after a second caudal block performed at the end of surgery.

without any signs of a neurologic pathology, perhaps in the context of an altered balance of the autonomic nervous system, and he has himself occasionally anisocoric pupils, especially when he is tired.

At the **lower extremity**, an unwanted epidural spread occasionally occurs with psoas compartment block (Schüpfer & Jöhr 2005). In addition, in the inguinal region the femoral nerve lies very superficial and can be blocked accidentally during ilioinguinal nerve block or wound infiltration (cf. Case 5.9).

Summary and Recommendations

This case illustrates the importance of ensuring that whenever local anaesthetic is injected at the head or the neck, no unwanted spread to the facial or vagal nerve occurs.

A Horner syndrome is a relatively common phenomenon, and it is usually recognized when only one side is affected. All caregivers have to be informed about the benign and transient nature of the phenomenon.

References

Aronson, L.A., Parker, G.C., Valley, R., *et al.* (2000). Acute Horner syndrome due to thoracic epidural analgesia in a paediatric patient. *Paediatr Anaesth*, 10, 89–91.

Courtman, S.P. & Carr, A.S. (2000). More Horner's than meets the eye. *Paediatr Anaesth*, 10, 455.

Hayek, G., Yazigi, A., Jebara, S., *et al.* (2003). Facial nerve paralysis during cervical plexus block for carotid artery endarterectomy. *J Cardiothorac Vasc Anesth*, 17, 782–783.

Jöhr, M. & Sossai, R. (1996). Facial nerve palsy after bat ear surgery. *Anesth Analg*, 83, 434.

Schiessler, R., Helmer, M., Kovarik, J., *et al.* (1989). Phrenic nerve block as a complication of local anesthetic infiltration for internal jugular vein catheterization. *Anesthesiology*, 71, 812–813.

Schüpfer, G. & Jöhr, M. (2005). Psoas compartment block in children: Part I: description of the technique. *Paediatr Anaesth*, 15, 461–464.

Silbert, J., Matta, N., Tian, J., *et al.* (2013). Pupil size and anisocoria in children measured by the plusoptiX photoscreener. *J AAPOS*, 17, 609–611.

Thermann, F., Ukkat, J., John, E., *et al.* (2007). Frequency of transient ipsilateral vocal cord paralysis in patients undergoing carotid endarterectomy under local anesthesia. *J Vasc Surg*, 46, 37–40.

Weksler, N., Nash, M., Rozentsveig, V., *et al.* (2001). Vocal cord paralysis as a consequence of peritonsillar infiltration with bupivacaine. *Acta Anaesthesiol Scand*, 45, 1042–1044.

Local Anaesthetic Toxicity

Case

Many years ago, a 2 3/12-year-old girl, weighing 12 kg, was brought to the children's hospital after a fall from a window. She was whimpering, restless, showed irregular breathing and had an obviously distorted thigh. After the administration of 15 μg of fentanyl a skin wheal in the inguinal region just lateral to the pulsating artery was made and a 25G insulated needle was inserted. The nerve stimulator was set at 1.0 mA with an impulse width of 0.1 ms. No twitches were elicited, but after a clear give the tip of the needle was thought to be below the fascia iliaca, and after careful aspiration 12 ml of a 1:1 mixture of levobupivacaine 0.5% and prilocaine 1% was injected (2.5 mg/kg levobupivacaine + 5 mg/kg prilocaine). Soon afterwards, the child appeared to be relaxed and repelled the approaching nurse with a decisive 'no'. The transfer to the CT scanner was prepared, but suddenly, 12 minutes after the injection, the child convulsed. The clonic convulsion subsided after administration of 20 mg of thiopental, and ventilation had to be briefly assisted with bag and mask. The decision was made to proceed with the spontaneously breathing but still unresponsive child to the CT scan for further diagnostics. The patient regained consciousness during transport. In addition to the femoral fracture, rib fractures and a small cerebral contusion area were found.

The femoral fracture was fixed by closed reduction and internal fixation under general endotracheal anaesthesia. Despite the positive-pressure ventilation and the presence of rib fractures, the team decided against inserting a chest tube because the thoracic region could be closely observed during the case. The child was extubated on table and the further course was uneventful.

Discussion

In this case the convulsions were likely to have been caused by **local anaesthetic toxicity**. The time delay of 12 minutes and the functioning analgesia from the femoral block indicate that rapid absorption and not a direct intravenous injection was responsible for the undesirably high plasma levels, although the doses used, with 2.5 mg/kg levobupivacaine, were in a high but still acceptable dose range. Prilocaine does not really add to toxicity, with the exception of generating methaemoglobin, which in this case was found to be at 3.6% after 90 minutes. Otherwise toxicity of mixtures of local anaesthetics is clearly additive; this has been shown for CNS toxicity as well as for cardiac toxicity. As no twitches could be elicited, the injection was probably made considerably lateral to the femoral nerve, similar to a fascia iliaca compartment block, below the fascia iliaca and probably always in part intramuscularly. When this block is performed with ropivacaine, a rapid absorption peaking as early as 10 minutes has been reported in children (Paut *et al.* 2004). As always, a diagnosis must be questioned: the coincidence of the small cerebral contusion and epilepsy would have been another possible explanation for the convulsions.

Local anaesthetic toxicity causes cerebral toxicity presenting with convulsions, and, more seriously, at higher doses cardiac toxicity. The **treatment** of **cerebral toxicity** consists in assuring oxygenation and interrupting convulsions by the administration of anticonvulsive compounds, e.g. benzodiazepines, thiopental or propofol. It has to be noted that a small dose of thiopental is usually sufficient to suppress convulsions; there is no need for a full induction dose, as for general anaesthesia followed by endotracheal intubation. In a case of severe **cardiac toxicity**, presenting with hypotension, conduction block and ventricular arrhythmias, the rules of advanced paediatric life support have to be followed; in particular, the administration of small doses of adrenaline is essential. In addition, lipid rescue is used, 1.5 ml/kg of lipid 20% followed by 15 ml/kg/h (Neal *et al.* 2012). The value of lipid rescue therapy has recently been questioned (Rosenberg 2016), but animal research as well as clinical cases underline its effectiveness (Weinberg 2017). Although the mechanism of action is still unknown, lipid rescue seems to play a major role in the treatment of the toxicity of local anaesthetics and other compounds (Presley & Chyka 2013).

Convulsions following the administration of local anaesthetics do occur; although in most cases CNS toxicity may be suppressed by the concomitantly administered general anaesthesia. In the famous first French ADARPEF study, including 24 409 regional blocks, two children convulsed (Giaufré *et al.* 1996). In the second ADARPEF study, including 31 132 regional blocks, 15 children showed signs of cardiac toxicity and one child convulsed in the group of 1262 pure regional blocks (Ecoffey *et al.* 2010). During his professional career the author was responsible for three cases in children, including the one described here. A school-aged girl convulsed during the injection of 1 ml/kg of 0.5% chloroprocaine for a Bier's block augmenting a partially failed distal sciatic nerve block. Obviously the tourniquet on the lower leg was not sufficiently tight. And ages ago, the author performed bilateral axillary plexus blocks for the reduction of both fractured forearms in an adolescent with a severe midface trauma. Plastic cannulas had been placed blindly into the perivascular sheath and 0.5% bupivacaine was given incrementally; because the blocks did not develop satisfactorily this ended up as 80 ml. Then the boy convulsed. This case occurred in the very early years of the use of bupivacaine, when doses up to 6–8 mg/kg were thought to be still safe.

A **femoral fracture** is a typical injury for a preschool child; the incidence peaks at the age of 2, when three times more boys than girls are involved (Bridgman & Wilson 2004). Paediatric femoral fracture is completely different to the adult type. A minimal trauma, e.g. a simple fall on the floor, is sufficient and blood loss is negligible (Lynch *et al.* 1996). Therefore providing analgesia is the first thing to do and fluid administration is usually not needed. On the scene, nasal fentanyl, e.g. 1.5 µg/kg, is a good option followed as soon as possible by a **femoral nerve block**. Femoral nerve block is the only major conduction block which can be indicated outside the hospital in emergency medicine (Ronchi *et al.* 1989). Over more than two decades it had been the standard practice in the children's hospital in Lucerne that every time a child with a suspected femoral fracture arrived, the anaesthetist was called to perform a femoral nerve block prior to removing the clothes and taking the x-ray. Unfortunately, because of new organizational structures, the enthusiasm to call a specialist has diminished.

Summary and Recommendations

This case illustrates that even with a correct technique, local anaesthetic toxicity is always with us as a possibility when we perform high-volume regional blocks; the necessary precautions have to be taken.

For the treatment of cerebral toxicity, maintaining adequate oxygenation and the administration of small doses of thiopental or propofol are sufficient to interrupt the convulsions.

For cardiac toxicity, small doses of adrenaline (e.g. 1 µg/kg) followed by lipid rescue (1.5 ml/kg lipid 20%) are recommended for supporting the circulation.

References

Bridgman, S. & Wilson, R. (2004). Epidemiology of femoral fractures in children in the West Midlands region of England 1991 to 2001. *J Bone Joint Surg Br*, 86, 1152–1157.

Ecoffey, C., Lacroix, F., Giaufré, E., *et al.* (2010). Epidemiology and morbidity of regional anesthesia in children: a follow-up one-year prospective survey of the French-Language Society of Paediatric Anaesthesiologists (ADARPEF). *Paediatr Anaesth*, 20, 1061–1069.

Giaufré, E., Dalens, B., & Gombert, A. (1996). Epidemiology and morbidity of regional anesthesia in children: a one-year prospective survey of the French-Language Society of Pediatric Anesthesiologists. *Anesth Analg*, 83, 904–912.

Lynch, J.M., Gardner, M.J., & Gains, B. (1996). Hemodynamic significance of pediatric femur fractures. *J Pediatr Surg*, 31, 1358–1361.

Neal, J.M., Mulroy, M.F., & Weinberg, G.L. (2012). American Society of Regional Anesthesia and Pain Medicine checklist for managing local anesthetic systemic toxicity: 2012 version. *Reg Anesth Pain Med*, 37, 16–18.

Paut, O., Schreiber, E., Lacroix, F., *et al.* (2004). High plasma ropivacaine concentrations after fascia iliaca compartment block in children. *Br J Anaesth*, 92, 416–418.

Presley, J.D. & Chyka, P.A. (2013). Intravenous lipid emulsion to reverse acute drug toxicity in pediatric patients. *Ann Pharmacother*, 47, 735–743.

Ronchi, L., Rosenbaum, D., Athouel, A., *et al.* (1989). Femoral nerve blockade in children using bupivacaine. *Anesthesiology*, 70, 622–624.

Rosenberg, P.H. (2016). Current evidence is not in support of lipid rescue therapy in local anaesthetic systemic toxicity. *Acta Anaesthesiol Scand*, 60, 1029–1032.

Weinberg, G. (2017). Current evidence supports use of lipid rescue therapy in local anaesthetic systemic toxicity. *Acta Anaesthesiol Scand*, 61, 365–368.

Case

5.5

Methaemoglobinaemia

Case

An 11-month-old girl, weighing 8 kg, tried to stand up with her hands on a wall mirror, which broke away and fell on her feet. The big toe was severely bruised, looking semi-amputated. She was brought to the children's hospital, where a surgical revision was indicated.

The anaesthetic plan was intravenous sedation plus a peripheral nerve block. After rectal premedication with midazolam 1 mg/kg, venous access was achieved, S-ketamine 3 mg/kg was administered in divided doses, and a popliteal sciatic nerve block was performed using a nerve stimulator. A volume of 0.9 ml/kg of a mixture containing prilocaine 1% and levobupivacaine 0.5% was injected. The block was obviously successful, because no further sedation was required. The girl slept quietly while protected with headphones from the noisy surroundings. The surgical intervention took 70 minutes. In the middle of the case, 1 hour after performing the block, the anaesthetist suddenly noticed that the oxygen saturation was gradually decreasing, and it ultimately reached 89% despite nasal oxygen administration.

Because there was no other symptom and the child was quietly breathing, the most probable diagnosis was methaemoglobinaemia, especially after the administration of prilocaine 4.5 mg/kg, which could have caused it. A blood sample was not taken, so as to avoid waking the child. 10 mg (1.1 mg/kg) of methylene blue was given by a slow intravenous injection. As expected (see below), oxygen saturation came down to 72% for a moment and then, over the next 15 minutes, increased to 97% without additional oxygen (Fig. 5.5).

The parents were informed about the event, which was an innocuous influence on saturation readings and not really a complication. In addition, they were warned to expect a blue coloration of all body fluids, easily visible in the nappies.

Discussion

This case illustrates that low saturation readings are not always due to pulmonary problems, but that a wider differential diagnosis is needed including elevated concentrations of **methaemoglobin (Met-Hb)**. The clinical picture of methaemoglobinaemia is a normally breathing child with no signs of cyanotic heart disease, but with a catastrophic appearance with a greyish-blue colour and a pulse oximeter reading of around 85%. Met-Hb is a derivative of the normal haemoglobin occurring when the Fe^{++} is oxidized to Fe^{+++}; it does not take part in the oxygen transport. The concentration of Met-Hb is normally below 1% of total haemoglobin. It is continuously formed, but immediately reduced by two enzymes.

One hour after
performing the block

During the injection
of methylene blue

10 minutes after
methylene blue

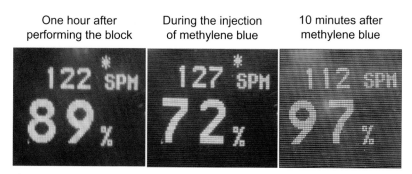

Figure 5.5 The pulse oximeter readings before, during and 10 minutes after the injection of methylene blue.

At 10% Met-Hb cyanosis is usually apparent, at 20% clinical symptoms appear, and a concentration of more than 50–70% may be rapidly fatal. Met-Hb influences pulse oximeter readings because it has a high absorption at the currently used wavelengths, 660 nm and 940 nm. When moderate concentrations are present, 2% Met-Hb reduces the reading of the pulse oximeter by 1%; high levels drive the reading towards 85%, independent of the actual concentration (Barker *et al.* 1989). Therefore, in the presence of Met-Hb, the real oxygen saturation is always lower than the indicated one. This means that when the oxygen saturation reading falls below 90%, the Met-Hb concentration should be measured. In this case, however, the decision was to proceed directly to treatment because taking a blood sample would have disturbed the smoothly running clinical process – and because modern multi-wave pulse oximetry was not yet available (Barker *et al.* 2006).

In the clinical surroundings, **methaemoglobinaemia** is most often induced by drugs increasing the oxidative stress to the haemoglobin. For the anaesthetist, local anaesthetics, the topical anaesthetic benzocaine, and especially prilocaine, which is converted to methyl-aniline (ortho-toluidine), are the most commonly incriminated compounds (Guay 2009). However, at high doses, lidocaine too has the potential to cause methaemoglobinaemia (Neuhaeuser *et al.* 2008). Because the enzyme Met-Hb reductase does not reach adult levels before 3 months of age, already moderate doses of prilocaine can cause relevant concentrations of Met-Hb (Frey & Kehrer 1999). Numerous cases have been reported after the application in preterm and term neonates; however, when the dose limits were followed, there was no case with a relevant elevation of the Met-Hb concentration (Guay 2009). This means restricting the application of EMLA to 1 g (one patch) applied on 10 cm² in the age group 0–2 months, and to 2 g in the age group 3–12 months. It was the author's practice, with good success, to restrict the dose of prilocaine to 5 mg/kg for nerve blocks in infants. This case shows that individual patients may be more vulnerable. Outside anaesthesia, antimicrobial agents, vasodilators and nitric oxide are commonly accused compounds. Occasionally, exposure to nitrate/nitrite compounds by the dietary route can also cause severe methaemoglobinaemia (Zeman *et al.* 2002). As a very rare exception, a congenital form with diminished enzyme activity or an unstable haemoglobin variant can be encountered.

Whereas moderately elevated concentrations of Met-Hb, e.g. up to 15–20%, present only a 'cosmetic problem' for a healthy infant, the margin of safety of the oxygen supply is reduced, and this may become relevant in children with cardiac or pulmonary diseases. Higher concentrations of Met-Hb require treatment, especially because Met-Hb leads in addition to a shift of the oxygen binding curve to the left (because of an increased affinity for oxygen in the remaining heme sites that are in the ferrous state within the same tetrameric haemoglobin unit). It was the author's practice to administer methylene blue to the few children who showed visible cyanosis, because it is difficult to convince nurses and parents that this type of cyanosis is benign and does not cause harm.

The **treatment** of choice is methylene blue 1 mg/kg intravenously, slowly injected over 5 minutes. Methylene blue acts as an electron carrier for NADPH-Met-Hb reductase: its normally insignificant activity is markedly increased and Met-Hb is rapidly reduced. Methylene blue is contraindicated in children with glucose-6-phosphate dehydrogenase deficiency, because with deficient NADPH regeneration it causes haemolytic anaemia. Rapid intravenous administration of methylene blue leads, as in this case, to transient spurious readings with pulse oximetry (Fig. 5.5), as long as a large part of the compound is in the pulsating arterial compartment of the circulation (Trillo & Aukburg 1992); as soon as the compound is equally distributed throughout the body, the readings come back to the baseline value.

Summary and Recommendations

This case illustrates that methaemoglobinaemia has to be taken into account when potentially incriminated drugs, such as prilocaine, have been used, even in only moderate doses.

It is wise to measure Met-Hb, even with methaemoglobinaemia of known origin, as soon as the oxygen saturation readings approach 90%. The treatment of choice is methylene blue 1 mg/kg, which causes during the injection a spurious dip in the saturation readings.

This story also illustrates that the decision for a treatment, in this case with methylene blue, should be based not only on objective numbers, but also has to include the feelings of the parents. It may not be acceptable for them to take their child home with a grossly cyanotic appearance.

References

Barker, S.J., Curry, J., Redford, D., et al. (2006). Measurement of carboxyhemoglobin and methemoglobin by pulse oximetry: a human volunteer study. *Anesthesiology*, 105, 892–897.

Barker, S.J., Tremper, K.K., & Hyatt, J. (1989). Effects of methemoglobinemia on pulse oximetry and mixed venous oximetry. *Anesthesiology*, 70, 112–117.

Frey, B. & Kehrer, B. (1999). Toxic methaemoglobin concentrations in premature infants after application of a prilocaine-containing cream and peridural prilocaine. *Eur J Pediatr*, 158, 785–788.

Guay, J. (2009). Methemoglobinemia related to local anesthetics: a summary of 242 episodes. *Anesth Analg*, 108, 837–845.

Neuhaeuser, C., Weigand, N., Schaaf, H., et al. (2008). Postoperative methemoglobinemia following infiltrative lidocaine administration for combined anesthesia in pediatric craniofacial surgery. *Paediatr Anaesth*, 18, 125–131.

Trillo, R.A. & Aukburg, S. (1992). Dapsone-induced methemoglobinemia and pulse oximetry. *Anesthesiology*, 77, 594–596.

Zeman, C.L., Kross, B., & Vlad, M. (2002). A nested case–control study of methemoglobinemia risk factors in children of Transylvania, Romania. *Environ Health Perspect*, 110, 817–822.

Total Spinal Anaesthesia

Case

Many years ago, a 4-year-old boy, weighing 15 kg, was scheduled for bilateral orchidopexy. After an inhalational induction a size 2.5 classic type laryngeal mask airway (LMA) was placed and the child breathed spontaneously a mixture of oxygen, air and halothane. A caudal block using a 25G butterfly needle was performed by a resident under direct supervision of the senior paediatric anaesthetist. A test dose of 3 ml (0.2 ml/kg) followed by 17 ml bupivacaine 0.125% with adrenaline 5 µg/ml was administered using repeated aspiration, as was standard practice in the institution. Afterwards the child was transferred from the induction room to the operating theatre.

About 30 minutes later, the senior paediatric anaesthetist supervising three theatres made his routine round. The resident was relaxed; he was ventilating the child manually, administering 0.25 V% halothane, and reported that the caudal worked perfectly and everything was stable. However, the institutional practice was to maintain spontaneous ventilation throughout the case; on questioning, the resident reported that about 15 minutes earlier he had started to assist ventilation because of progressively shallow breathing. As this was an unexpected finding in a child breathing 1/3 MAC of a halogenated agent who had not received any opioid, the suspicion arose that this could signify a high spinal block. The pupils were medium-sized and unreactive to light. Transcutaneous tetanic stimulation at 60 mA applied to the upper extremity provoked massive muscle contractions by direct stimulation but not the slightest increase in heart rate.

As surgery proceeded on the second side, approximately 90 minutes after the caudal injection, slight diaphragmatic movements could be seen; spontaneous ventilation returned and the LMA was removed by the end of surgery. The legs were still flaccid, the child was pain-free, but the arms showed only sloppy uncontrolled movements.

Discussion

This case of **total spinal anaesthesia** following an accidental intrathecal injection during a caudal block stresses several educational points.

First, the **incidence** of an accidental total spinal block during attempted caudal epidural block is low; therefore it is not expected by the practitioner and a modest backflow of cerebrospinal fluid through the thin cannula with extension tubing may not be present or may be overlooked. In the author's institution caudal blocks have been performed since 1984, with an annual frequency of over 600 blocks initially and then coming down to 400 annual blocks because of the increasing popularity of peripheral nerve blocks. Looking at the experience of more than three decades, a total spinal block occurred in about 1:1500 caudal blocks. With one exception, they all presented in a non-dramatic way, like the presented case, and were often difficult to recognize. The exception was a 3 kg neonate who very rapidly developed apnoea and arterial hypotension; ironically this block was performed under ultrasound guidance in a teaching situation; an epidural spread could not be observed, and the bubbling appearance of the subarachnoid space was seen but not interpreted correctly. In the literature the incidence of recognized total spinal block following an attempted caudal injection is low; in a retrospective series of 236 caudal blocks there was one total spinal block (Hoelzle *et al.* 2010). Dural taps have been reported in 1:1415 (Ecoffey *et al.* 2010) or in 1:1250 (Suresh *et al.* 2015) caudal blocks.

Second, the **clinical signs** are sometimes very subtle in an anaesthetized child with a secured airway and controlled ventilation. In the spontaneously breathing child, progressively shallow breathing is a typical sign, but all the other symptoms have to be actively sought: unresponsiveness to pain in the upper part of the body and pupils which are unreactive to light. Because the sympathetic and parasympathetic supplies are blocked, both pupils are often medium-sized and not maximally dilated. Transcutaneous tetanic electrical stimulation, using a nerve stimulator designed for monitoring neuromuscular blockade, allows reliable detection of the reaction to pain, because, in clinical doses, inhalational agents alone do not completely suppress the cardiovascular reaction to pain (Zbinden *et al.* 1994). The **speed of onset** as well as the duration of such an event is often overestimated. In adults isobaric spinal anaesthesia using bupivacaine shows a rather slow onset and the block extension is at its maximum only after 30–60 minutes (Tuominen 1991). In paediatric patients too, block extension was found to be maximal at 45 minutes after the intrathecal injection of 0.5 mg/kg isobaric bupivacaine in children 2–5 years of age (Kokki *et al.* 1992). On the other hand the duration of analgesia was limited to 75 minutes. In the patient described here the dose was 25 mg (1.66 mg/kg) bupivacaine, which is much higher than the highest recommended dose for spinal anaesthesia in the literature, 0.7 mg/kg for this age group. Nevertheless, in the anaesthetized child, the progression to a total spinal block can be overlooked, and by the end of a longer case spontaneous ventilation has usually resumed.

Third, **haemodynamic stability** is reasonably maintained even during a high spinal block. But, in contrast to the classic assumption that hypotension is absent after neuraxial anaesthesia in preschool children, in reality this is not the case, especially when the block is performed under general anaesthesia (Jöhr & Berger 2012). Especially in neonates and young infants, hypotension is regularly seen when a neuraxial block is performed in addition to general anaesthesia (McCann *et al.* 2017). Nevertheless, a cardiovascular collapse leading to cardiac arrest, which is the major threat of total spinal anaesthesia in the adult geriatric population, never happens in children.

Total spinal anaesthesia can also occur during **planned spinal anaesthesia** and when recommended doses are used. In a series of 339 spinal anaesthetics, eight high spinal blocks occurred (Hoelzle *et al.* 2010). Especially with hyperbaric spinal anaesthesia, changes of position have to be done very carefully after the intrathecal injection. Between 1987 and 2003, the author used spinal anaesthesia extensively for inguinal hernia repair in former preterm infants using hyperbaric tetracaine and adrenaline; on a few occasions assisted ventilation was needed for a short time, but a total spinal block never occurred. With **psoas compartment block** an accidental intrathecal injection can also occur, and the child has to be monitored closely (Schüpfer & Jöhr 2005).

The **prevention** of an accidental total spinal block is a meticulous technique; in the very tiny baby and in case of a suspected anomaly, a short look with the ultrasound probe where the dural sac ends is always worthwhile. In addition, the needle should never be inserted too deeply in the sacral canal (Adewale *et al.* 2000), a few millimetres beyond the sacrococcygeal membrane is sufficient in order to avoid a dural tap.

Summary and Recommendations

This case shows that accidental high spinal anaesthesia can occur after attempted caudal epidural anaesthesia.

As a total spinal block can evolve quite slowly, a child should be under close supervision for at least 30 minutes.

A meticulous technique is helpful to avoid an accidental dural puncture; unfortunately, clinical experience tells us that even the use of ultrasound does not absolutely guarantee that it will never happen.

References

Adewale, L., Dearlove, O., Wilson, B., *et al.* (2000). The caudal canal in children: a study using magnetic resonance imaging. *Paediatr Anaesth*, 10, 137–141.

Ecoffey, C., Lacroix, F., Giaufré, E., *et al.* (2010). Epidemiology and morbidity of regional anesthesia in children: a follow-up one-year prospective survey of the French-Language Society of Paediatric Anaesthesiologists (ADARPEF). *Paediatr Anaesth*, 20, 1061–1069.

Hoelzle, M., Weiss, M., Dillier, C., *et al.* (2010). Comparison of awake spinal with awake caudal anesthesia in preterm and ex-preterm infants for herniotomy. *Paediatr Anaesth*, 20, 620–624.

Jöhr, M. & Berger, T.M. (2012). Caudal blocks. *Paediatr Anaesth*, 22, 44–50.

Kokki, H., Hendolin, H., Vainio, J., *et al.* (1992). Pediatric surgery: a comparison of spinal anesthesia and general anesthesia [in German]. *Anaesthesist*, 41, 765–768.

McCann, M.E., Withington, D.E., Arnup, S.J., *et al.* (2017). Differences in blood pressure in infants after general anesthesia compared to awake regional anesthesia (GAS study: a prospective randomized trial). *Anesth Analg*, 125, 837–845.

Schüpfer, G. & Jöhr, M. (2005). Psoas compartment block in children: Part I: description of the technique. *Paediatr Anaesth*, 15, 461–464.

Suresh, S., Long, J., Birmingham, P.K., *et al.* (2015). Are caudal blocks for pain control safe in children? An analysis of 18,650 caudal blocks from the Pediatric Regional Anesthesia Network (PRAN) database. *Anesth Analg*, 120, 151–156.

Tuominen, M. (1991). Bupivacaine spinal anaesthesia. *Acta Anaesthesiol Scand*, 35, 1–10.

Zbinden, A.M., Petersen-Felix, S., & Thomson, D.A. (1994). Anesthetic depth defined using multiple noxious stimuli during isoflurane/oxygen anesthesia. II. Hemodynamic responses. *Anesthesiology*, 80, 261–267.

Case

Many years ago, a 12-year-old girl, 36 kg, was scheduled for bilateral osteotomies of both the distal femur and the distal tibia. After an inhalational induction a size 3 laryngeal mask airway (LMA) Supreme was placed and the child breathed spontaneously while femoral nerve blocks as well as proximal dorsal sciatic nerve blocks were performed on both sides, using a total of 46 ml of 0.25% bupivacaine with clonidine 1.5 µg/ml. Then the child was ventilated and paralysed by a continuous infusion of mivacurium. Haemodynamic stability was maintained with a mean arterial pressure at around 50 mmHg over the 5-hour procedure. Only moderate bleeding occurred, and in addition to Ringer's lactate 500 ml of a starch solution was administered.

In the afternoon, after skin closure, the girl emerged smoothly and completely pain-free and was transferred directly to the ward where she stayed with her parents. About an hour later the anaesthetist made his postoperative pain round before leaving the hospital. 500 ml of Ringer's lactate had been given because of marginally low blood pressure. The patient was pale but comfortable, and there was no visible bleeding, but one leg was obviously much colder than the other. No pulsations of the tibial or fibular artery could be felt in that leg.

The anaesthetist informed the responsible orthopaedic surgeon face to face about a potentially serious vascular problem. At revision surgery, a surgical sectioning of the proximal part of the popliteal artery was found at the height of the femoral osteotomy. The continuity of the popliteal artery was reconstructed, and fasciotomy of the anterior tibial compartment was performed. The further course included multiple interventions for further fasciotomies, debridement and vascular revisions. The severe compartment syndrome, with creatine kinase (CK) concentrations of more than 29000 U/l, the completely deranged coagulation system, generalized oedema and a serious pain problem necessitated a stay on the ICU for several weeks.

Although it was the anaesthetist who was responsible for the timely diagnosis, this case prompted a lively discussion in the hospital on the role of regional blocks in orthopaedic surgery.

Discussion

This case of severe **compartment syndrome** following a corrective osteotomy leading to a partial loss of function of the lower limb illustrates the importance of good postoperative surveillance. In this case, a direct surgical trauma to the arterial supply led to ischaemia, swelling and rhabdomyolysis. There is a vivid discussion in the literature about the danger of masking compartment syndromes by long-lasting regional blocks (Ivani *et al.* 2015), but the conclusions are equivocal. With neuraxial blockades, especially with epidural analgesia, breakthrough pain is still possible (Mar *et al.* 2009), whereas with continuous peripheral blocks it may be difficult (Munk-Andersen & Laustrup 2013, Walker *et al.* 2012), and with a dense peripheral block it is surely impossible. Because the early warning signs such as paraesthesia, pain, especially on passive movement, loss of sensation and paralysis are obscured, only the very late signs such as absent arterial pulse and increased muscle tightness are present. A high index of suspicion is needed, and if there is any doubt the compartment pressure must be measured (Staudt *et al.* 2008); this can be done without pain in the presence of a still functioning peripheral block, but otherwise deep sedation or general anaesthesia is required. Normal values of compartment pressure are slightly higher in children than in adults, but a value over 30 mmHg is nevertheless an indication for intervention.

In the author's opinion, postoperative **regional blocks** have the potential to mask a compartment syndrome; however, the fact that these patients are closely observed by an additional team, the anaesthetic pain service, may largely outweigh this negative aspect. In this particular case it was the anaesthetist who was responsible for the timely diagnosis.

For the **prevention** of problems it is important to select the technique, the drug and the concentration very carefully, for every individual child. For example, for the closed reduction of a tibial fracture a caudal block using 0.2% ropivacaine may be preferable to a combined femoral and sciatic nerve block. The caudal block could also be done with a mixture of 1% prilocaine and 0.2% ropivacaine in order to have a dense block of short duration but still some analgesia. A femoral nerve block alone will never mask a compartment syndrome, and therefore it can be done with long-lasting and highly concentrated compounds, whereas the accompanying sciatic block may often be better performed with less concentrated solutions or a shorter-acting drug.

The anaesthetist must be familiar with the typical **situations at risk** (Fig. 5.7): tibial fractures (Shore *et al.* 2013), compression trauma of the forefoot (Bibbo *et al.* 2000) and closed reduction and internal fixation of forearm fractures (Martus *et al.* 2013).

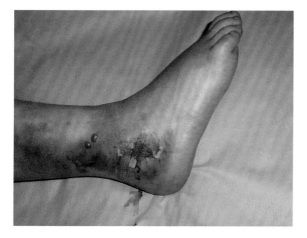

Figure 5.7 In this other child with an ankle fracture and massive swelling a fasciotomy was indicated.

Summary and Recommendations

Regional blocks have theoretically the potential to mask an evolving compartment syndrome, and a high index of suspicion is needed.

If in doubt, the compartment pressure must be measured, and a value over 30 mmHg should trigger further investigations and treatment.

References

Bibbo, C., Lin, S.S., & Cunningham, F.J. (2000). Acute traumatic compartment syndrome of the foot in children. *Pediatr Emerg Care*, 16, 244–248.

Ivani, G., Suresh, S., Ecoffey, C., *et al.* (2015). The European Society of Regional Anaesthesia and Pain Therapy and the American Society of Regional Anesthesia and Pain Medicine Joint Committee practice advisory on controversial topics in pediatric regional anesthesia. *Reg Anesth Pain Med*, 40, 526–532.

Mar, G.J., Barrington, M.J., & McGuirk, B.R. (2009). Acute compartment syndrome of the lower limb and the effect of postoperative analgesia on diagnosis. *Br J Anaesth*, 102, 3–11.

Martus, J.E., Preston, R.K., Schoenecker, J.G., *et al.* (2013). Complications and outcomes of diaphyseal forearm fracture intramedullary nailing: a comparison of pediatric and adolescent age groups. *J Pediatr Orthop*, 33, 598–607.

Munk-Andersen, H. & Laustrup, T.K. (2013). Compartment syndrome diagnosed in due time by breakthrough pain despite continuous peripheral nerve block. *Acta Anaesthesiol Scand*, 57, 1328–1330.

Shore, B.J., Glotzbecker, M.P., Zurakowski, D., *et al.* (2013). Acute compartment syndrome in children and teenagers with tibial shaft fractures: incidence and multivariable risk factors. *J Orthop Trauma*, 27, 616–621.

Staudt, J.M., Smeulders, M.J., & van der Horst, C.M. (2008). Normal compartment pressures of the lower leg in children. *J Bone Joint Surg Br*, 90, 215–219.

Walker, B.J., Noonan, K.J., & Bösenberg, A.T. (2012). Evolving compartment syndrome not masked by a continuous peripheral nerve block: evidence-based case management. *Reg Anesth Pain Med*, 37, 393–397.

Ischaemic Extremity

Case

Many years ago, a 2 10/12-year-old girl, weighing 17 kg, presented at the children's hospital with a dislocated distal humeral fracture. Circulation was maintained, but tingling fingers were reported. Anaesthesia was induced with 125 mg (7 mg/kg) thiopental, 35 μg (2 μg/kg) fentanyl and 10 mg (0.6 mg/kg) rocuronium. The trachea was intubated with a size 5.0 uncuffed endotracheal tube and anaesthesia maintained with sevoflurane.

After speedy closed reduction and percutaneous fixation of the fracture the surgeon wanted to apply the cast, but then he realized that the forearm felt cold and the radial pulse was absent. Using a Doppler device, no signal could be found distal to the elbow. After a brief discussion the decision was made to follow the anaesthetist's suggestion of first trying the effects of a plexus block on the vascular bed before proceeding to revision surgery.

Using a nerve stimulator, an axillary brachial plexus block was performed using 14 ml bupivacaine 0.25%. Five minutes later a radial pulse could be detected with the Doppler device, and 15 minutes later strong radial and ulnar pulses were felt. The further post-operative course was uneventful.

Discussion

This case shows that **avoiding regional anaesthesia** for fear of disguising neurologic damage caused by trauma or surgery, and of subsequently being involved in discussions on the causal relationships of a neurologic deficit, may not be in the best interest of the patient. It had been the institutional policy to provide a regional block to every such trauma patient in order to achieve good postoperative pain relief. But in this individual child the anaesthesia team avoided a regional block because of the history of tingling fingers. But, realistically, even if the tingling had persisted after reduction of the fracture, early surgical revision of the median and ulnar nerves would never have been an option. The only possible course of action would have been to exclude a compartment syndrome (cf. Case 5.7) or vascular damage.

The suggestion to avoid regional anaesthesia in the case of a **pre-existing neurologic deficit** is marginally supported by the theoretical risk that a second injury to a nerve fibre may worsen the functional outcome. However, there are no clinical data to support this theory. The cause of a nerve injury following peripheral nerve blockade is often multi-factorial, including needle trauma, compression and ischaemia, neurotoxicity and inflam-mation (Brull *et al.* 2015). It is probable that none of these factors is more likely to occur when there is a pre-existing neurologic deficit. Nerve injury is relatively common after elbow surgery (Kopp *et al.* 2015), but a brachial plexus block does not increase the risk of postoperative ulnar neuropathy after ulnar nerve transposition because of pre-existing neurologic problems (Hebl *et al.* 2001). Therefore, from this point of view, using a plexus block from the start to provide postoperative analgesia would have been an option.

The mechanisms behind **vascular insufficiency** following an elbow fracture (Fig. 5.8) include vasospasm, thrombosis following an intima tear, and a complete disruption of the artery. For the first of these, vasodilatation is a therapeutic option, but for the latter two the only option is surgery. Peripheral and central nerve blocks provide vasodilatation by blocking the sympathetic fibres. Their effectiveness in reversing vasospasm has been demonstrated in hand surgery (Audenaert *et al.* 1991), vascular catheterization (Breschan *et al.* 2004), chemical irritation (Kessell & Barker 1996) and regional blockade (Kaplanian *et al.* 2007). In adults a 400% increase in brachial arterial blood flow was observed after a brachial plexus block (Mouquet *et al.* 1989), which enhances the success rate of a reliably functioning arteriovenous shunt. The same mechanism underlies the fact that digital nerve block can restore pulse oximeter signal detection (Bourke & Grayson 1991). The author remembers an infant in whom a failed femoral vein puncture with potential arterial puncture led to a white and pulseless leg; the application of a caudal block restored a well-perfused and pink leg (cf. Case 4.6).

In the presented case the radial pulse reappeared after the reduction of the fracture and the blockade of the sympathetic fibres supporting vasoconstriction. If the hand stays pink, but the radial pulse remains absent, a surgical revision is usually indicated.

Summary and Recommendations

This case illustrates that a regional block not only provides pain relief, but also protects against ischaemic complications, as long as vasospasm and not disruption of the vessel is the cause.

Withholding a regional block for 'legal reasons' may not be in the best interest of the patient.

In case of suspected vasospasm, a regional block providing vasodilatation is well worth a trial.

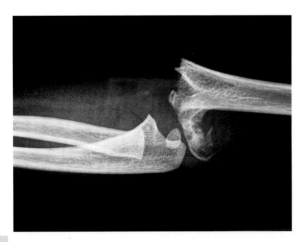

Figure 5.8 Dislocated supracondylar fracture, stretching vessels and nerves in the extreme.

References

Audenaert, S.M., Vickers, H., & Burgess, R.C. (1991). Axillary block for vascular insufficiency after repair of radial club hands in an infant. *Anesthesiology*, 74, 368–370.

Bourke, D.L. & Grayson, R.F. (1991). Digital nerve blocks can restore pulse oximeter signal detection. *Anesth Analg*, 73, 815–817.

Breschan, C., Kraschl, R., Jost, R., *et al.* (2004). Axillary brachial plexus block for treatment of severe forearm ischemia after arterial cannulation in an extremely low birth-weight infant. *Paediatr Anaesth*, 14, 681–684.

Brull, R., Hadzic, A., Reina, M.A., *et al.* (2015). Pathophysiology and etiology of nerve injury following peripheral nerve blockade. *Reg Anesth Pain Med*, 40, 479–490.

Hebl, J.R., Horlocker, T.T., Sorenson, E.J., *et al.* (2001). Regional anesthesia does not increase the risk of postoperative neuropathy in patients undergoing ulnar nerve transposition. *Anesth Analg*, 93, 1606–1611.

Kaplanian, S., Chambers, N.A., & Forsyth, I. (2007). Caudal anaesthesia as a treatment for penile ischaemia following circumcision. *Anaesthesia*, 62, 741–743.

Kessell, G. & Barker, I. (1996). Leg ischaemia in an infant following accidental intra-arterial administration of atracurium treated with caudal anaesthesia. *Anaesthesia*, 51, 1154–1156.

Kopp, S.L., Jacob, A.K., & Hebl, J.R. (2015). Regional anesthesia in patients with preexisting neurologic disease. *Reg Anesth Pain Med*, 40, 467–478.

Mouquet, C., Bitker, M.O., Bailliart, O., *et al.* (1989). Anesthesia for creation of a forearm fistula in patients with endstage renal failure. *Anesthesiology*, 70, 909–914.

Case

Decades ago, a 14-year-old boy, weighing 40 kg, was scheduled for spermatic vein ligation. After an intravenous induction with propofol the airway was secured with a size 3 laryngeal mask airway (LMA) and the child breathed spontaneously a mixture of oxygen, nitrous oxide and sevoflurane. An ilioinguinal nerve block was performed using a 30 mm long 22G subcutaneous needle, which was inserted in a line between the anterior superior iliac spine (ASIS) and the umbilicus, 2 cm medial to the ASIS, until a fascial give was thought to be felt. After careful aspiration, a total of 30 ml of a mixture of 0.25% bupivacaine and 1% prilocaine was injected, partially below the fascia followed by an extensive subcutaneous infiltration.

When the surgeon exposed the spermatic vein with a high inguinal incision, a dark bluish structure was seen shining through the peritoneal sac. The surgeon opened the peritoneum and found a small laceration of the colon and a subserous haematoma. The apparently non-perforating puncture was secured with a suture and the peritoneum was closed. The further course was uneventful. On postoperative day 5 the boy presented again because of discharge from the incision site, and this was managed conservatively. Six weeks later, because of persistent wound tenderness (Fig. 5.9), a surgical revision was done. This showed chronic inflammatory changes of the subcutaneous tissue, and the culture was positive for *Staphylococcus aureus*. Three days later, because of signs of acute inflammation, a third surgical intervention was performed; however, no abscess or fistula formation could be found. With wound drainage and antibiotic treatment the boy made a slow but complete recovery.

Discussion

This case of **colonic puncture during ilioinguinal nerve block**, which has been reported in part elsewhere (Jöhr & Sossai 1999), emphasizes that blind blocks of the abdominal wall carry an inherent risk of **abdominal wall perforation**. Puncturing visceral organs has been reported with ilioinguinal nerve block (Amory *et al.* 2003, Frigon *et al.* 2006), as well as with transverse abdominal plane (TAP) block (Long *et al.* 2014), and there is no doubt that rectus sheath block is associated with the identical risk. In addition, an **unwanted extension** of the blockade can occur. Using a landmark-based technique the needle tip was found to be in the correct place in only 14% of cases (Weintraud *et al.* 2008), and spread down to the femoral nerve can occur (Rosario *et al.* 1997). With a blind technique an incidence of leg weakness consistent with femoral nerve block greater than 5% has been reported both in adults (Ghani *et al.* 2002) and in children (Lipp *et al.* 2004). Even wound infiltration carried

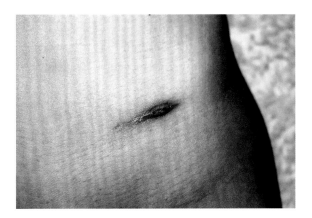

Figure 5.9 Delayed healing and chronic infection following an inguinal incision.

out by the surgeon for inguinal hernia repair has led to unwanted femoral nerve block and postoperative falls. Therefore, from the perspective of today, abdominal wall blocks should only be performed under ultrasound guidance.

Is there a **causal relationship** between the block performed and the infectious complication? With ilioinguinal nerve block the author has experienced intestinal punctures on two other occasions, and in both cases a greenish fluid containing small particles could be aspirated but no sequelae occurred. Puncturing the small bowel probably carries a minimal risk of infectious complications, causing problems only when the injection is made into the intestinal wall (Amory *et al.* 2003). Even in the presented case, with a purely superficial wound infection with *Staphylococcus aureus*, a causal relationship was not clearly established between the apparently non-perforating serosa laceration and the disturbed healing process; however, from the start, knowledge of the event caused uncertainty and perhaps triggered more extensive revision surgery.

The **type of needle** used can be questioned. A thin sharp needle, like the one used in this case, glides easily through the tissue, and today, with the use of ultrasound, gains more and more advocates. With a non-cutting short-bevelled needle (Plexufix type) the resistance of fascial structures can be felt more easily, and, theoretically, it seems to be more difficult to puncture a movable neural or visceral structure; on the other hand, more force has to be applied to advance the needle, which is potentially more traumatic. In at least two cases of a small bowel haematoma such a needle had been used (Amory *et al.* 2003, Frigon *et al.* 2006).

The **choice of the anaesthetic technique** for lower abdominal incisions is a matter of debate (Aveline *et al.* 2011, Fredrickson *et al.* 2010). Ilioinguinal nerve block is widely used for inguinal hernia repair and orchidopexy; TAP block provides reliable analgesia covering the segments T10 to T12 and has a good safety record (Long *et al.* 2014). Today, an ultrasound-guided TAP block would be the preferred choice for an open appendectomy or a spermatic vein ligation. In the author's opinion it is the preferred technique for inguinal hernia repair too, as it is effective and a clear ultrasound image can reliably be obtained.

Summary and Recommendations

This case shows that abdominal wall blocks inherently carry the risk of abdominal wall perforation and intestinal puncture. Therefore, today, these blocks should exclusively be performed under ultrasound guidance.

While injecting local anaesthetics in the inguinal region under ultrasound guidance, a spread down to the femoral nerve has to be carefully avoided.

This case also illustrates that, even when probably no causally related damage occurs, an unwanted event may have a negative influence on the further postoperative treatment.

References

Amory, C., Mariscal, A., Guyot, E., et al. (2003). Is ilioinguinal/iliohypogastric nerve block always totally safe in children? *Paediatr Anaesth*, 13, 164–166.

Aveline, C., Le, H.H., Le, R.A., et al. (2011). Comparison between ultrasound-guided transversus abdominis plane and conventional ilioinguinal/iliohypogastric nerve blocks for day-case open inguinal hernia repair. *Br J Anaesth*, 106, 380–386.

Fredrickson, M.J., Paine, C., & Hamill, J. (2010). Improved analgesia with the ilioinguinal block compared to the transversus abdominis plane block after pediatric inguinal surgery: a prospective randomized trial. *Paediatr Anaesth*, 20, 1022–1027.

Frigon, C., Mai, R., Valois-Gomez, T., et al. (2006). Bowel hematoma following an iliohypogastric-ilioinguinal nerve block. *Paediatr Anaesth*, 16, 993–996.

Ghani, K.R., McMillan, R., & Paterson-Brown, S. (2002). Transient femoral nerve palsy following ilio-inguinal nerve blockade for day case inguinal hernia repair. *J R Coll Surg Edinb*, 47, 626–629.

Jöhr, M. & Sossai, R. (1999). Colonic puncture during ilioinguinal nerve block in a child. *Anesth Analg*, 88, 1051–1052.

Lipp, A.K., Woodcock, J., Hensman, B., et al. (2004). Leg weakness is a complication of ilio-inguinal nerve block in children. *Br J Anaesth*, 92, 273–274.

Long, J.B., Birmingham, P.K., De Oliveira, G.S.J., et al. (2014). Transversus abdominis plane block in children: a multicenter safety analysis of 1994 cases from the PRAN (Pediatric Regional Anesthesia Network) database. *Anesth Analg*, 119, 395–399.

Rosario, D.J., Jacob, S., Luntley, J., et al. (1997). Mechanism of femoral nerve palsy complicating percutaneous ilioinguinal field block. *Br J Anaesth*, 78, 314–316.

Weintraud, M., Marhofer, P., Bösenberg, A., et al. (2008). Ilioinguinal/iliohypogastric blocks in children: where do we administer the local anesthetic without direct visualization? *Anesth Analg*, 106, 89–93.

Complications of Caudal Anaesthesia

Case

Many years ago, a 2 8/12-year-old boy, weighing 14 kg, was scheduled for unilateral orchidopexy. After an inhalational induction the airway was secured with a size 2.0 laryngeal mask airway (LMA) Supreme and the child breathed spontaneously a mixture of oxygen, air and sevoflurane. Following standard procedure in the institution, the boy was placed in the left lateral position for a caudal block, the upper hip flexed 90°, the lower one 45°. The palpation of the anatomical landmarks, especially of the sacral cornua, was a little confusing but it was possible to guess the correct site for needle insertion. The supervising senior paediatric anaesthetist was for a brief moment inattentive, and then he suddenly realized that the resident, who was already advanced in his training, had inserted the 30 mm long 25G needle with a 32° Crawford bevel (Epican Paed) down to the hub. The resident remarked that he was continuously advancing the needle while expecting the give at the perforation of the sacrococcygeal membrane.

It was immediately clear that this needle, almost perpendicular to the skin, was inserted far too deeply. The drapes were removed and a careful digital rectal examination revealed the needle projecting at least 1 cm from the anterior surface of the sacrum, stretching the apparently still intact mucosa in a tent-like fashion.

The needle was carefully withdrawn and a single dose of cefuroxime 50 mg/kg was given prophylactically. Caudal block was abandoned and an ilioinguinal nerve block was performed for postoperative analgesia. The further course was uneventful, with no signs of local or systemic infection occurring.

Discussion

This case of **rectal puncture** during **attempted caudal block** illustrates that even unimaginable events can happen, when the ability of the practitioner to think in three dimensions is overstretched and landmarks are scarcely palpable, e.g. in an obese child. Two rectal punctures were reported in a large retrospective series including 158 229 caudal blocks (Gunter 1991), and in the ADARPEF study, which included 12 111 caudal blocks, one was seen (Giaufré *et al.* 1996). In addition, several case reports address this topic (Sathianathan & Dobby 2015, Varghese *et al.* 2016). In the presented case the **diagnosis** was made by visual imagination and digital rectal examination; in others, fluid seeped out of the anus during the injection or on repeated aspiration, never at the first aspiration, or fluid with faecal admixture could be aspirated (Sathianathan & Dobby 2015, Varghese *et al.* 2016).

Concerning **therapy**, in our case the barrier of the rectal mucosa had not definitely been pierced, although the findings of the digital examination were impressive, and an antibiotic was given as single shot. In the published cases a needle contaminated with stool was withdrawn and potentially deposited germs in the bone and the epidural space, so prolonged antibiotic coverage was indicated.

Overall, caudal epidural block is an extremely safe technique (Jöhr & Berger 2012). Complications can occur, but, to the author's knowledge, there is not a single reported case worldwide of permanent **neurologic damage** caused by epidural haematoma or epidural infection (Ecoffey *et al.* 2010, Giaufré *et al.* 1996, Gunter 1991, Suresh *et al.* 2015), despite the fact that millions of paediatric caudal blocks have been performed.

Infection is theoretically always a threat, but with a single-shot technique it should be a very rare event. In the only published case of sacral osteomyelitis following caudal block a debatable medication for skin disinfection was used, a watery solution of octenidine (Wittum *et al.* 2003). All other published infectious or technical complications occurred in the context of continuous catheter techniques. Nevertheless, a high hygienic standard is mandatory. Before palpating the landmarks the region should be swabbed in a craniocaudal direction with a 70% alcohol solution in order to reduce the amount of bacteria. Extensive skin disinfection with an alcoholic solution, sterile drapes and wearing sterile gloves should be the standard for every neuraxial blockade.

Local anaesthetic toxicity is best avoided by using an adrenaline-containing test dose and a slow and careful injection; repeated aspiration alone cannot reliably prevent an intravascular injection; in 6 out of 1100 caudal blocks the intravascular injection only became evident after the tachycardia caused by the adrenaline (Veyckemans *et al.* 1992). Severe toxicity also occurred, when too high a concentration was accidentally used, e.g. ropivacaine 0.75% instead of 0.2% (Ecoffey *et al.* 2010).

An **undesired block extension**, such as an insufficient or unilateral block, can occur. Intraoperatively, unilateral block is only recognized when the side of the surgery is affected. Postoperatively, the coughing or crying baby shows an asymmetrical abdomen, with the abdominal wall flaccid and bulging on the blocked side but not on the opposite side (Fig. 5.10). An accidental intrathecal injection can lead to a total spinal block (cf. Case 5.6).

A rare side effect is **self-limited back pain**; in a study focusing specifically on this problem an incidence of 4.7% has been reported (Valois *et al.* 2010). But in the author's institution, where all patients are followed up by telephone the day after surgery, back pain

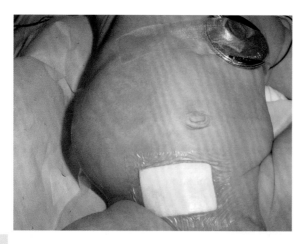

Figure 5.10 Postoperatively, the unilateral blockade is clearly visible by a flaccid abdomen on the blocked and a tight one on the non-blocked side.

was never mentioned, even after thousands of caudal blocks. Maybe the routine administration of NSAIDs to almost all our patients for postoperative analgesia is sufficient to blunt this local irritation.

Summary and Recommendations

This case of rectal puncture during attempted caudal block emphasizes that the insertion of a needle into the body is a physical injury and is always dangerous. It has to be planned and performed in a perfect and well-controlled way.

Otherwise, provided that an appropriate technique is used, caudal anaesthesia has a very good safety record.

This story also emphasizes that supervising trainees requires 100% attention throughout the procedure; it is only the presence of a fully attentive teacher that gives the trainee the necessary security and protection against complications.

References

Ecoffey, C., Lacroix, F., Giaufré, E., et al. (2010). Epidemiology and morbidity of regional anesthesia in children: a follow-up one-year prospective survey of the French-Language Society of Paediatric Anaesthesiologists (ADARPEF). Paediatr Anaesth, 20, 1061–1069.

Giaufré, E., Dalens, B., & Gombert, A. (1996). Epidemiology and morbidity of regional anesthesia in children: a one-year prospective survey of the French-Language Society of Pediatric Anesthesiologists. Anesth Analg, 83, 904–912.

Gunter, J. (1991). Caudal anesthesia in children: a survey. Anesthesiology, 75, A936.

Jöhr, M. & Berger, T.M. (2012). Caudal blocks. Paediatr Anaesth, 22, 44–50.

Sathianathan, V. & Dobby, N. (2015). Rectal puncture complicating caudal blockade in a child with severe rectal distension. Paediatr Anaesth, 25, 1063–1065.

Suresh, S., Long, J., Birmingham, P.K., et al. (2015). Are caudal blocks for pain control safe in children? An analysis of 18,650 caudal blocks from the Pediatric Regional Anesthesia Network (PRAN) database. Anesth Analg, 120, 151–156.

Valois, T., Otis, A., Ranger, M., et al. (2010). Incidence of self-limiting back pain in children following caudal blockade: an exploratory study. Paediatr Anaesth, 20, 844–850.

Varghese, N., Joseph, N., & Kandavar, S. (2016). Rectal puncture during caudal anaesthesia. Indian J Anaesth, 60, 371–372.

Veyckemans, F., Van Obbergh, L.J., & Gouverneur, J.M. (1992). Lessons from 1100 pediatric caudal blocks in a teaching hospital. Reg Anesth, 17, 119–125.

Wittum, S., Hofer, C.K., Rolli, U., et al. (2003). Sacral osteomyelitis after single-shot epidural anesthesia via the caudal approach in a child. Anesthesiology, 99, 503–505.

6 Medication-Related Problems

Medication Error

Case 6.1

Case

A long time ago, a 2 8/12-year-old girl, 14 kg, was scheduled for full-body scintigraphy because of suspected osteomyelitis in the presence of recurrent febrile episodes. The intention was to induce sedation with propofol 15 mg (1 mg/kg) and ketamine 10 mg (0.7 mg/kg). The anaesthetist injected 1.5 ml of milky solution, which was propofol, and 1 ml from a syringe with a green label, typical for racemic ketamine at the time.

Shortly after the injection, gurgling respiration and upper airway obstruction occurred, followed by apnoea. For the skilled anaesthetist, mask ventilation was easy and uneventful, but soon afterwards a reddish skin rash became visible. Because the whole episode was unclear for the team, the author was informed. Apnoea and skin rash are typical signs of a rapid injection of atracurium, and because at least two similar cases had occurred in his own practice, the diagnosis of a confusion between atracurium and ketamine (both with a green label) was made by phone.

A laryngeal mask airway (LMA) size 2 was inserted and the child was ventilated with oxygen and nitrous oxide; two additional doses of propofol were given for sedation. At the end of the examination the residual neuromuscular block was antagonized with neostigmine 50 μg/kg combined with glycopyrrolate 10 μg/kg. The girl made a completely uneventful recovery and the parents were informed about the event.

Discussion

This case illustrates a classic **medication error**, confounding two compounds with a labelling of similar colour ('lookalikes'). Many of the recognized medication errors concern muscle relaxants, because the apnoea makes it immediately obvious that something has gone wrong. In contrast, other errors are often initially overlooked, e.g. profound sedation caused by an incorrect concentration of a hypnotic (S-ketamine 25 mg/ml instead of 5 mg/ml), tachycardia because of ephedrine instead of thiopental 10 mg/ml (both in a 5 ml syringe), increased diuresis because of furosemide instead of metamizole (lookalike vials). During his professional career the author witnessed or himself made many medication errors.

A major step forward was the introduction of **colour-coded labelling** in many but not all countries (Balzer *et al.* 2012). Muscle relaxants now have a red label (Fig. 6.1), and confusion between two different relaxants has not had the same impact as the administration of a relaxant instead of a hypnotic agent, as in the presented case.

The institution has to be made **resilient against errors**, which will always occur. The most catastrophic medication errors are flushing an intravenous line with potassium

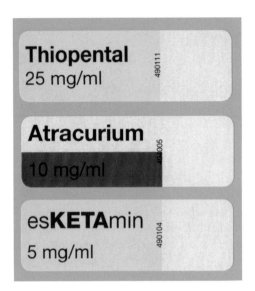

Figure 6.1 Colour-coded labels have greatly increased safety, but thiopental is still occasionally injected instead of S-ketamine.

chloride instead of normal saline. The use of the wrong concentration of a local anaesthetic, e.g. ropivacaine 0.75% instead of 0.2% for a caudal block, can induce a toxic reaction (Hübler *et al.* 2010). In oncology patients, the deadly intrathecal injection of vincristine instead of methotrexate is an ever-present threat (Liu *et al.* 2017). Special precautions have to be taken to avoid these disasters and to make the working surrounding resilient against mistakes by an individual staff member. For example, in the children's hospital in Lucerne no potassium vials are kept in stock in the operating theatres; if needed, potassium has to be ordered from the ward. Only ropivacaine 0.2% is available in the children's hospital, and levobupivacaine 0.5% has to be used for more dense blocks. The author is convinced that in paediatric anaesthesia a muscle relaxant has always to be ready in a syringe for immediate injection. This means that it needs to be stored on the anaesthesia trolley in a dedicated place in order to avoid confusion with other medication (Martin *et al.* 2017). For neuraxial anaesthesia and in oncology, non-Luer connectors are intended to be introduced, in order to avoid the intrathecal injection of a compound exclusively suited for intravenous injection (Lawton *et al.* 2009).

Special attention is needed when verbal orders are given to staff not necessarily familiar with the medication they are told to inject. The culture of **closed-loop communication**, to repeat what was heard, has to be both taught and practised (Davis *et al.* 2017).

Dosing errors are a typical issue in paediatrics. Because of the hundredfold difference in body weight between a preterm baby and an adolescent, no single dose size can be remembered by the practitioner. In adults half to one ampoule of many drugs may be correct, but in paediatrics the dose has to be calculated for every individual child. **Electronic prescribing** systems have the potential to reduce such errors on the ward and in intensive care settings (Jani *et al.* 2010), and at the children's hospital such an electronic system has been running successfully for almost a decade. However, they are probably not suitable for the busy surroundings of the operating room. Dosing errors by **a factor of 10** do occur; this has been reported to occur once a week in a large paediatric institution (Doherty & McDonnell 2012). The author has twice observed nalbuphine dosed at 10 mg instead of

1 mg; fortunately, nalbuphine is a compound with a large margin of safety and high doses are well tolerated even by small babies (Schultz-Machata *et al.* 2014).

Summary and Recommendations

This case illustrates a medication error, confusing a relaxant and a hypnotic compound, which probably occurred because of the similar colour of the labels.

The introduction of colour coding has reduced the severity of confusion, because a drug of the same class is administered. However, continuous care and clear communication remain the cornerstones of safe practice.

The anaesthesia workplace has to be made resilient against mistakes. Confusions with immediately lethal consequences, e.g. potassium instead of normal saline for flushing, are best avoided by physically eliminating certain compounds from the busy theatre workplace.

References

Balzer, F., Wickboldt, N., Spies, C., *et al.* (2012). Standardised drug labelling in intensive care: results of an international survey among ESICM members. *Intensive Care Med*, 38, 1298–1305.

Davis, W.A., Jones, S., Crowell-Kuhnberg, A.M., *et al.* (2017). Operative team communication during simulated emergencies: too busy to respond? *Surgery*, 161, 1348–1356.

Doherty, C. & McDonnell, C. (2012). Tenfold medication errors: 5 years' experience at a university-affiliated pediatric hospital. *Pediatrics*, 129, 916–924.

Hübler, M., Gäbler, R., Ehm, B., *et al.* (2010). Successful resuscitation following ropivacaine-induced systemic toxicity in a neonate. *Anaesthesia*, 65, 1137–1140.

Jani, Y.H., Barber, N., & Wong, I.C. (2010). Paediatric dosing errors before and after electronic prescribing. *Qual Saf Health Care*, 19, 337–340.

Lawton, R., Gardner, P., Green, B., *et al.* (2009). An engineered solution to the maladministration of spinal injections. *Qual Saf Health Care*, 18, 492–495.

Liu, H., Tariq, R., Liu, G.L., *et al.* (2017). Inadvertent intrathecal injections and best practice management. *Acta Anaesthesiol Scand*, 61, 11–22.

Martin, L.D., Grigg, E.B., Verma, S., *et al.* (2017). Outcomes of a failure mode and effects analysis for medication errors in pediatric anesthesia. *Paediatr Anaesth*, 27, 571–580.

Schultz-Machata, A.M., Becke, K., & Weiss, M. (2014). Nalbuphine in pediatric anesthesia [in German]. *Anaesthesist*, 63, 135–143.

Drug Overdose

Case

A 7-month-old girl, weighing 8 kg, was scheduled for surgical release of a tethered cord. The paediatric anaesthetist went to the neurosurgical unit. Anaesthesia was induced by mask; after achieving venous access, nasotracheal intubation was performed. The further instrumentation included an additional venous access; an arterial line and a bladder catheter were inserted. During this preparation phase and the placement of the leads for monitoring the motor and sensory evoked potentials, haemodynamic stability was well maintained.

In order to enhance the registration of evoked potentials, the decision was made to switch from the inhalational to a total intravenous technique. The anaesthetist instructed the assistant to start the propofol perfusor at a rate of 80 mg per hour (10 mg/kg/h) and sevoflurane was switched off. In addition, remifentanil was started at the rate of 0.1 µg/kg/min. A few minutes later mean arterial pressure had dropped close to 30 mmHg, and the BIS monitor showed a flat EEG tracing which predominantly showed the electrocardiographic spikes of the QRS complex (Fig. 6.2). At this point it was noticed that the propofol perfusor was running at a rate of 80 ml per hour instead of 8 ml per hour, which would have corresponded to the desired 80 mg per hour. Propofol administration was stopped for more than 20 minutes until the EEG had recovered from isoelectric to regular activity. The further course was uneventful.

Discussion

This is a typical **failure in communication** leading to a 10-fold error in dosing propofol (Doherty & McDonnell 2012). It is part of a good safety culture to dose medication always in milligrams (mg) or micrograms (µg) and not in millilitres (ml). Even more correct would have been to say '80 milligrams per hour, this equals 8 millilitres per hour'. In addition, a closed-loop communication is recommended, which means that the recipient repeats the information as heard, which is then confirmed. Medication errors, especially errors in dosing, are much more common in paediatric practice than in adults because there is no 'usual dose' in view of the body weight varying from 500 g to 130 kg (Kaufmann *et al.* 2017). In adults one or half an ampoule rarely causes major harm if it is not a vial designated to be admixed to an infusion: in children this is definitively not the case.

This neurosurgical intervention was performed outside the paediatric hospital, and therefore the paediatric anaesthetist was working in strange surroundings with personnel not used to paediatric patients. In such a situation, good **team performance** cannot be taken for granted, and a clear closed-loop communication style, always reconfirming the message,

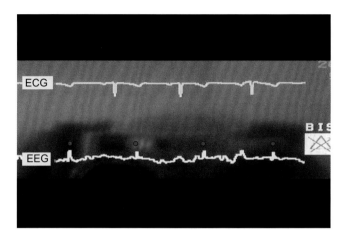

Figure 6.2 An EEG tracing showing an isoelectric EEG in a child; this is not obvious at first glance, but when the ECG signal is visible in the EEG, this is usually the case.

is even more important than it is in the paediatric hospital, where everybody is familiar with paediatric doses and nobody would infuse 100 mg/kg/h of propofol to a child. The same problem occurs when new and unfamiliar drugs are used: the author remembers a very similar event with a rapidly administered overdose of dexmedetomidine, 20 ml instead of 20 μg, which led to profound bradycardia and hypertension in a sick child.

Dosing errors are probably more common with **total intravenous anaesthesia** than with inhalational anaesthesia, especially when using ordinary infusion pumps for the propofol administration (Pandit *et al.* 2014). Pumps are switched off for transfer and erroneously not restarted in theatre, which can lead to unwanted intraoperative awareness; or, as in this case, a 10-fold overdose can happen. Very likely the use of **target-controlled infusion** (TCI) would have avoided this event. Although the Paedfusor system is only recommended in children over 1 year of age, it can be used in infants too, and, in the author's opinion, it is advantageous because it is still safer than a manually driven pump. TCI increases safety because it eliminates the errors that can typically be made in manual systems (Schnider *et al.* 2016). It provides a constant plasma level of propofol by administering a bolus followed by a gradually decreasing infusion. The TCI models are not very precise in predicting the exact height of the plasma concentration and they do not tell us at all if this concentration corresponds to the clinical needs of the patient. Nevertheless, a manually driven infusion never performs better than a TCI pump. In the author's hands the Schnider model (Schnider *et al.* 1998) is well suited to children older than 5 years (Rigouzzo *et al.* 2010); below this age the Paedfusor (Marsh *et al.* 1991) or the Kataria (Kataria *et al.* 1994) model should be used.

EEG-based monitoring, e.g. BIS or Narcotrend, should be used whenever possible during total intravenous anaesthesia in order to have some kind of pharmacodynamic feedback (Louvet *et al.* 2016). The primary goal is not avoidance of awareness, but optimizing dosing; in this case a flat EEG first raised the suspicions of the anaesthetist. Both a massive overdose leading to a flat EEG, and a failing administration because of paravenous infusion or a failing pump can be detected with the aid of these devices – even though, in children below 1 year of age, the EEG cannot be reliably used to guide hypnosis during general anaesthesia (Hayashi *et al.* 2012).

Summary and Recommendations

This case of a 10-fold overdose of propofol during total intravenous anaesthesia illustrates the importance of clear communication.

Target-controlled infusion (TCI) increases safety because typical errors are avoided.

During total intravenous anaesthesia, EEG-based monitoring is helpful to recognize an overdose or a failing drug administration.

As part of safety culture, the dose of a medication should always be quoted in weight units (μg, mg or g) and additionally in volumes (ml).

References

Doherty, C. & McDonnell, C. (2012). Tenfold medication errors: 5 years' experience at a university-affiliated pediatric hospital. *Pediatrics*, 129, 916–924.

Hayashi, K., Shigemi, K., & Sawa, T. (2012). Neonatal electroencephalography shows low sensitivity to anesthesia. *Neurosci Lett*, 517, 87–91.

Kataria, B.K., Ved, S.A., Nicodemus, H.F., *et al.* (1994). The pharmacokinetics of propofol in children using three different data analysis approaches. *Anesthesiology*, 80, 104–122.

Kaufmann, J., Wolf, A.R., Becke, K., *et al.* (2017). Drug safety in paediatric anaesthesia. *Br J Anaesth*, 118, 670–679.

Louvet, N., Rigouzzo, A., Sabourdin, N., *et al.* (2016). Bispectral index under propofol anesthesia in children: a comparative randomized study between TIVA and TCI. *Paediatr Anaesth*, 26, 899–908.

Marsh, B., White, M., Morton, N., *et al.* (1991). Pharmacokinetic model driven infusion of propofol in children. *Br J Anaesth*, 67, 41–48.

Pandit, J.J., Andrade, J., Bogod, D.G., *et al.* (2014). 5th National Audit Project (NAP5) on accidental awareness during general anaesthesia: summary of main findings and risk factors. *Br J Anaesth*, 113, 549–559.

Rigouzzo, A., Servin, F., & Constant, I. (2010). Pharmacokinetic-pharmacodynamic modeling of propofol in children. *Anesthesiology*, 113, 343–352.

Schnider, T.W., Minto, C.F., Gambus, P.L., *et al.* (1998). The influence of method of administration and covariates on the pharmacokinetics of propofol in adult volunteers. *Anesthesiology*, 88, 1170–1182.

Schnider, T.W., Minto, C.F., Struys, M.M., *et al.* (2016). The safety of target-controlled infusions. *Anesth Analg*, 122, 79–85.

Inadvertent Drug Administration

Case

A school class visited the children's hospital in order to learn a bit about medicine and the hospital environment. The pupils, aged 7–9 years, had a look at some surgical instruments, they were shown how a cast was put on to one of them, and finally they were shown an anaesthesia induction room. An anaesthetist and an anaesthetic nurse demonstrated the anaesthesia machine and the monitoring devices. The most adventurous girl placed herself on the operating table, so that the monitoring could be demonstrated: a blood pressure cuff was put on her arm, and the ECG and pulse oximeter probe were placed. By now she already looked pretty nervous. A flavoured face mask was given to her to be placed over her mouth and nose with the aim of demonstrating the capnographic tracing. She got even more nervous and started to breathe deeply, showed jerky movements, and finally became unresponsive. The anaesthetist tried to calm her, because he was convinced that what he was observing was a hyperventilation episode in a young girl. He placed her in lateral position on a stretcher and explained the episode to the upset class and the anxious teacher. Within 10 minutes the girl made an uneventful recovery without nausea and vomiting. The school class left the children's hospital, the girl with the stigma of being a little bit special.

Later in the afternoon the sevoflurane vaporizer was found to be set at 4 V% (Fig. 6.3). So the girl had just accidentally received a sevoflurane anaesthetic.

Discussion

This case of **inadvertent drug administration** is just a spectacular presentation of a common phenomenon. The vaporizer is still set at high concentrations of the inhalational agents, whereas the fresh gas is turned off. The next user just turns on the fresh gas and places the mask on the patient's face, e.g. in order to preoxygenate. The author remembers numerous cases occurring at induction of anaesthesia, when the child rejected the mask because of the smell of the inhalational agent. Similarly nitrous oxide is sometimes accidentally given, because some devices have a simple switch for deciding between air and nitrous oxide, and the gas no longer has to be dosed by a rotameter. The author has been called several times because a patient did not wake up and the only reason was the continuing administration of nitrous oxide. The author wonders that the industry has not yet made changes in a way that the fresh gas supply can only be turned off when the vaporizer is closed, and it is surprising that even some modern anaesthesia workstations can be switched off with an open vaporizer.

A similar type of error is leaving open the fresh gas supply, usually oxygen, after the termination of anaesthesia. Flushing a circle system over many hours, typically over a

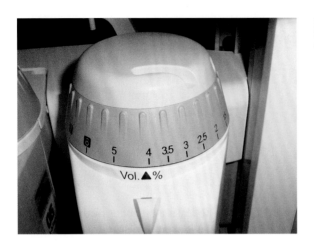

Figure 6.3 The vaporizer is left open, and instead of pure oxygen the child receives 4% sevoflurane.

weekend, leads to a completely **desiccated absorbent**. Desiccated absorbent reacts in a different way with inhalational agents. This leads to the degradation of the inhalational agent in an **exothermic reaction** with increased formation of carbon monoxide and other degradation products (Wissing *et al.* 2001). Whereas with desflurane it is mainly carbon monoxide production that is in the focus of interest, with sevoflurane the absorbent can reach temperatures of several hundred degrees Celsius and compounds irritating the airway are formed (Wissing *et al.* 1997). The author remembers a 3-year-old girl who was the first case on a Monday morning. She was induced by mask with sevoflurane and nitrous oxide and went to sleep, then the nitrous oxide was turned off. One minute later she suddenly began to cough, sat up and pushed the mask away and was fully awake with a still irritated airway. The absorbent canister was extremely hot. It was clear that sevoflurane had been reaching the patient at first, but then with increasing temperature sevoflurane was degraded in the absorbent canister before it could reach the patient. As the phenomenon was already known from the literature, early diagnosis was made, and it could be reconstructed that oxygen was indeed already turned on, when the circuit check was made. In the late 1990s this led to a change of practice such that the fresh gas supply was always detached from the wall connectors over the weekend. Happily this type of complication is no longer possible with modern anaesthesia workstations, because switching off the device automatically stops the oxygen supply.

The **accumulation of carbon monoxide** with reduced fresh gas flow, even with a correctly hydrated absorbent, has been discussed in the past. There are mainly three sources for the elevated concentration of carbon monoxide haemoglobin: the degradation of sevoflurane, parental (or, rarely in children, the patient's) smoking, and haemoglobin breakdown.

Accidentally administering anaesthesia to a healthy schoolgirl visiting the hospital is a delicate affair, and careful and timely **communication** is recommended. It is wise and correct to inform the accompanying teacher as well as the parents about the event, telling them what happened, that we are sorry, and, most important, that there will be no long-term sequelae. However, in the presented case, even the anaesthetist did not immediately check what was going on and the open vaporizer was only detected afterwards. It has been the author's practice to call parents down to the operating suite whenever something unexpected and unwanted has happened, e.g. a massive extravasation, in order to ensure that it is brought to the parents' notice immediately and they do not first hear about it afterwards from the nurses. Parents usually do not complain because a complication happened, but because they were not immediately and fully informed.

Summary and Recommendations

Before placing the mask on the patient's face it must be checked that only the desired gases are administered. There is no excuse for negligence.

Desiccated absorbent, which occurs after an expanded dry gas flow, enhances the breakdown of halogenated agents and has to be replaced.

In case of an inadvertent event, it is of paramount importance that the parents are informed in a timely and personal, face-to-face manner, in order to retain their confidence.

References

Wissing, H., Kuhn, I., & Dudziak, R. (1997). Heat production from reaction of inhalation anesthetics with dry soda lime [in German]. *Anaesthesist*, 46, 1064–1070.

Wissing, H., Kuhn, I., Warnken, U., *et al.* (2001). Carbon monoxide production from desflurane, enflurane, halothane, isoflurane, and sevoflurane with dry soda lime. *Anesthesiology*, 95, 1205–1212.

Drug Administration during Total Intravenous Anaesthesia

Case

Many years ago, a 2-week-old girl, born at 23 3/7 weeks of gestation, weighing 640 g, was scheduled for emergency laparotomy because of intestinal perforation. Following the institutional practice, surgery was performed in the neonatal intensive care unit (NICU) and the neonatal ventilator was used. The anaesthetic regime was based on a high-dose opioid technique: a total of 120 μg/kg fentanyl and 0.2 mg/kg pancuronium was administered over the 3-hour procedure. During surgery, which included the insertion of a Broviac catheter, small bowel resection and ileostomy, 20 ml/kg of packed red cells and 10 ml/kg of fresh frozen plasma were given in addition to crystalloids. The baby remained remarkably stable, and the only vasopressor needed was dopamine up to 5 μg/kg/min.

Forty-seven hours later duct ligation was indicated. The intention was again to administer pancuronium and fentanyl. At the arrival of the anaesthetist the mean arterial pressure was high, at 55 mmHg; pancuronium and fentanyl were given, the dopamine infusion was turned off, and the baby was positioned for surgery. There was no reaction to skin incision and surgery proceeded as planned. But at the end of the case, when the drapes were removed, the anaesthetist broke out in a sweat when he suddenly noticed that the three-way-stopcock was in a position which impeded the administration of fentanyl (Fig. 6.4a).

Discussion

This case illustrates that **failed drug administration** is an inherent risk of every total intravenous technique. In this case the three-way stopcock was turned to the wrong position; other pitfalls include infiltrated lines, disconnected tubing (Fig. 6.4b), leaking syringes, failing pumps and, most important, the anaesthetist simply making a mistake. The author has painfully experienced all these situations. Therefore all these potential failures have to be excluded before starting the case and the specific sites have to be checked repeatedly throughout the case. However, in neonatal surgery access to the patient is very limited. A failure in the administration of propofol, e.g. the pump is turned off and not restarted, is a common cause of awareness (Pandit *et al.* 2014). In addition, some kind of pharmacodynamic feedback is recommended, e.g. an EEG-based monitor (Constant & Sabourdin 2012); but the EEG can only reliably be used for monitoring the depth of hypnosis in children older than 1 year.

In this 640 g baby, for the initial operation a **high-dose opioid** anaesthetic was used. There is no consensus about the optimal anaesthetic technique for this type of patient. They are usually dependent on a neonatal ventilator with no possibility of administering

(a)

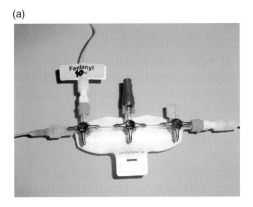

Figure 6.4a A three-way stopcock in the wrong position impeded the administration of fentanyl.

(b)

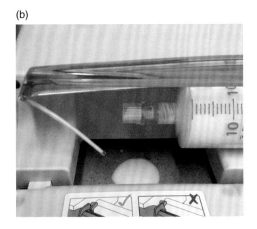

Figure 6.4b Interrupted administration of propofol because of defective tubing in another patient.

inhalational agents, and the only option is an intravenous technique. Two questions need to be answered: the necessary dose for sufficient analgesia and the need for a hypnotic.

First, for these extremely preterm patients there are no data about the necessary **dosage**. Some practitioners use moderate doses of morphine, e.g. 250 µg/kg – but maybe sufficient analgesia is only mimicked because the hypotensive side effect impedes the increase in blood pressure at skin incision. Experts recommend a dose of 25 µg/kg fentanyl for duct ligation (Wolf 2012). In a pharmacokinetic study, 30 µg/kg fentanyl resulted in haemodynamic stability at skin incision but not at the time of skin closure (Collins *et al.* 1985). In slightly older babies a dose of 25–50 µg/kg resulted in haemodynamic stability during sternotomy (Duncan *et al.* 2000). Remifentanil is rarely used in this context; 1 µg/kg/min suppresses the haemodynamic and hormonal stress response (Weale *et al.* 2004). Traditionally the author used a dose of at least 50 µg/kg fentanyl given as a short infusion over 5–10 minutes, always preceded by a muscle relaxant, in order to avoid rigor with the inability to ventilate the patient (Fahnenstich *et al.* 2000). For the second intervention, this patient erroneously did not receive any fentanyl at all because the three-way stopcock was turned to the wrong position, but nevertheless haemodynamic stability during surgery was maintained. How can this be explained? A very long elimination half-time of between 6 and 32 hours has been reported in preterm babies with a gestational age between 23 and 38 weeks

(Collins *et al.* 1985). Therefore, 47 hours after the extremely high dose of 120 µg/kg fentanyl, plasma levels may still have been sufficient to blunt the haemodynamic stress response.

Second, there is a debate on the necessity of **amnesia and hypnosis** as part of the anaesthetic regime in this age group. There is no doubt that profound analgesia and the absence of dyspnoea are essential. But, as long as no fear about the future exists, at least up to the age when stranger anxiety is common, sleep and amnesia are probably not necessarily needed and a pure opioid regime is defensible. If an awake regional technique were used, no one would request sleep and amnesia. This is further underlined by the fact that even at early school age, where intraoperative awareness is a relatively common complication of general anaesthesia (Davidson *et al.* 2011), being accidentally awake during surgery does not provoke anxiety and long-term sequelae to the extent that it does in adults (Phelan *et al.* 2009). As long as children live in their 'magic world' and unexplained perceptions are a normal part of their lives, they are protected against the negative consequences of being awake. A hypnotic agent is therefore not essential for neonatal anaesthesia; nonetheless, it has to be admitted that traces of sevoflurane markedly increase haemodynamic stability at the time of skin incision.

This case of **major surgery in a small patient** also prompts a discussion on the need for placing central venous and arterial catheters. Reliable venous access is essential. The question will always be what we can get with an acceptable risk in a 640 g baby. The author aimed for at least one line with backflow; in this case it was a surgically implanted Broviac catheter into the internal jugular vein, placed before beginning laparotomy. Because of his own negative experiences, the author strongly recommends doing this in two steps: first the Broviac catheter, then remove the drapes and connect the line, before positioning and preparing for laparotomy.

Summary and Recommendations

Failed drug administration is an inherent risk of total intravenous anaesthesia. Meticulous care is needed to avoid all technical drawbacks.

A pharmacodynamic feedback system, e.g. EEG-based monitoring, should be standard practice in children above 1 year of age.

This case also illustrates the unsolved debate about the optimal anaesthetic regime in very tiny babies. A high-dose opioid regime is often used e.g. for duct ligation.

Vascular access with backflow, which allows taking blood samples, is recommended for major surgery in small babies.

References

Collins, C., Koren, G., Crean, P., *et al.* (1985). Fentanyl pharmacokinetics and hemodynamic effects in preterm infants during ligation of patent ductus arteriosus. *Anesth Analg*, 64, 1078–1080.

Constant, I. & Sabourdin, N. (2012). The EEG signal: a window on the cortical brain activity. *Paediatr Anaesth*, 22, 539–552.

Davidson, A.J., Smith, K.R., Blusse van Oud-Alblas, H.J., *et al.* (2011). Awareness in children: a secondary analysis of five cohort studies. *Anaesthesia*, 66, 446–454.

Duncan, H.P., Cloote, A., Weir, P.M., *et al.* (2000). Reducing stress responses in the pre-bypass phase of open heart surgery in infants and young children: a comparison of different fentanyl doses. *Br J Anaesth*, 84, 556–564.

Fahnenstich, H., Steffan, J., Kau, N., *et al.* (2000). Fentanyl-induced chest wall rigidity and laryngospasm in preterm and term infants. *Crit Care Med*, 28, 836–839.

Pandit, J.J., Andrade, J., Bogod, D.G., *et al.* (2014). 5th National Audit Project (NAP5) on accidental awareness during general anaesthesia: summary of main findings and risk factors. *Br J Anaesth*, 113, 549–559.

Phelan, L., Stargatt, R., & Davidson, A.J. (2009). Long-term posttraumatic effects of intraoperative awareness in children. *Paediatr Anaesth*, 19, 1152–1156.

Weale, N.K., Rogers, C.A., Cooper, R., *et al.* (2004). Effect of remifentanil infusion rate on stress response to the pre-bypass phase of paediatric cardiac surgery. *Br J Anaesth*, 92, 187–194.

Wolf, A.R. (2012). Ductal ligation in the very low-birth weight infant: simple anesthesia or extreme art? *Paediatr Anaesth*, 22, 558–563.

Propofol Infusion Syndrome

Case

Many years ago, a 5-year-old boy, weighing 17 kg, was scheduled for an occipital craniotomy and medulloblastoma resection in the prone position. Some days earlier, propofol-based sedation for an MRI had been uneventful. After an inhalational induction with sevoflurane a total intravenous technique with propofol and remifentanil was chosen in order to allow reliable registration of the evoked potentials; these were traditionally recorded by a specialized neuroanaesthetist in this institution. The further instrumentation, beside peripheral venous access and a size 5.0 cuffed nasotracheal tube, included a radial arterial line, a central venous catheter via the right internal jugular vein, a BIS monitor and a bladder catheter. The anaesthetic course was uneventful over 8 hours, haemodynamic stability was maintained, and no vasoactive support was needed. At the end of the case the body temperature was 36.5 °C. The regularly taken blood gases were within the normal range. But shortly after arrival in the paediatric intensive care unit (PICU) a metabolic acidosis with an elevated lactate concentration of 4.8 mmol/l was evident; the lactate concentration peaked soon afterwards at 7 mmol/l and was accompanied by a creatine kinase (CK) of 480 U/l. Over the next few hours the values gradually returned to normal. The presumptive diagnosis of a propofol infusion syndrome was made. Propofol had been infused at a rate of 10 mg/kg/h over 6 hours.

Some weeks later radiation therapy was initiated, with daily sessions over several weeks. Now the question arose: was it safe, with such a history, to administer daily propofol?

Discussion

This case shows that **propofol infusion syndrome (PRIS)** is always a threat when propofol is administered over a prolonged time. PRIS was initially described in the early 1990s, with a high mortality after prolonged administration of propofol to children in the intensive care setting (Parke *et al.* 1992). But PRIS also occurs in the context of anaesthesia of duration as short as 150 minutes (Kill *et al.* 2003, Mehta *et al.* 1999).

The **pathophysiology** is only partly understood; mitochondrial toxicity is clearly a prime suspect (Krajcova *et al.* 2015). At the beginning of the century, based on a case report (Wolf *et al.* 2001), impaired oxidation of fatty acids was postulated (Vasile *et al.* 2003). The mitochondrial oxidative metabolism is blocked; propofol impedes the electron flow through the respiratory chain and interacts with coenzyme Q (Vanlander *et al.* 2015); propofol is thus mimicking a 'pseudohypoxic state'. This lack of energy at a cellular level induces rhabdomyolysis, hyperkalaemia and cardiac pump failure with bradycardia and a Brugada type ECG. In addition, the cardiac toxicity is enhanced by high concentrations of

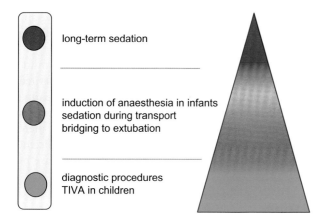

long-term sedation

induction of anaesthesia in infants
sedation during transport
bridging to extubation

diagnostic procedures
TIVA in children

Figure 6.5 Recommendations for the clinical use of propofol in children in the author's institution, using the traffic light analogy (red, unwise; amber, debatable; green, widely accepted).

free fatty acids. The body has recourse to anaerobic metabolism, and therefore metabolic acidosis and increasing lactate levels are early signs of PRIS (Koch *et al.* 2004). At an early stage these changes are reversible when the propofol administration is stopped or reduced (Koch *et al.* 2004); as it progresses, fatalities are common. A great number of cases have been reported, affecting both children and adults, during intensive care and during anaesthesia. PRIS can occur even at doses below 4 mg/kg/h (Krajcova *et al.* 2015).

For several reasons the occurrence of PRIS is more obvious in **children**. First, for pharmacokinetic reasons children need very high doses of propofol to achieve a sufficient depth of sedation or anaesthesia. Second, the high metabolic rate combined with the limited glycogen stores induces an early recurrence to fatty acid oxidation. Third, children are usually otherwise healthy, and mortality of cardiac origin should rarely occur in a child sedated and ventilated because of a respiratory infection. So the singularity of the symptoms of PRIS makes diagnosis relatively easy; whereas the elderly multimorbid adult patient often has many other reasons for circulatory failure, and cardiac death and the diagnosis of PRIS is probably often overlooked.

PRIS is an established entity **in adults**; in otherwise healthy subjects 10% mortality was caused by propofol in head-injured patients (Cremer *et al.* 2001) or patients with refractory status epilepticus (Iyer *et al.* 2009). With high doses of propofol, 35% of these patients showed signs of PRIS. PRIS is not just a rare idiosyncratic event; it is more likely a dose-dependent phenomenon which could even affect a majority of our patients, although some individuals may be more sensitive.

In some reported cases the propofol infusion was stopped for several hours, and then restarted at a low infusion rate; early after **re-exposure**, PRIS developed. Therefore, in the case described here, the safety of daily propofol administration over several weeks for radiation therapy was questioned. As there was no answer in the scientific literature, the pragmatic approach was to proceed with propofol for these daily short anaesthetics and to measure blood gas and lactate at the end of the first week, which showed ensuring normal values.

Propofol is in wide **clinical use** in paediatric anaesthesia. Pain at injection, hypotension and bradycardia are typical complications and are regularly seen. PRIS is a rarer event, but, including this case, the author has seen three cases of PRIS during his professional career. In addition, several times rumours about severe or even lethal cases reached him.

A grass-green discoloration of the urine is another rare side effect of propofol, but it seems to be benign and not to indicate a patient at increased risk of developing PRIS. The author's recommendations for the clinical use of propofol are summarized in Fig. 6.5.

Virtually all anaesthetic agents, not only propofol, have a depressant effect on mitochondrial energy production. In **mitochondrial disorders**, a group of rare inherited neurologic/metabolic disorders often presenting with myopathy and/or encephalopathy, deficient energy production similar to PRIS seems to be causal, and therefore some experts recommend avoiding propofol in such patients and using volatile agents instead. But there is no proof that this is relevant; we could also argue that something that is already deficient cannot be blocked by propofol. Nevertheless the precision in dosing favours the use of inhalational agents anyway.

Summary and Recommendations

This case illustrates that propofol infusion syndrome (PRIS) is an inherent risk of prolonged propofol administration in children and adults.

Propofol must not be given over a prolonged period of time. No reliable information can be given to answer the question, 'how long is too long?'

During prolonged anaesthetics, e.g. more than 3 hours, controlling lactate concentrations will probably allow a timely diagnosis of an evolving PRIS.

The history of PRIS also shows that it can take almost two decades until the majority of the practitioners are aware of a potentially life-threatening iatrogenic complication.

References

Cremer, O.L., Moons, K.G., Bouman, E.A., *et al.* (2001). Long-term propofol infusion and cardiac failure in adult head-injured patients. *Lancet*, 357, 117–118.

Iyer, V.N., Hoel, R., & Rabinstein, A.A. (2009). Propofol infusion syndrome in patients with refractory status epilepticus: an 11-year clinical experience. *Crit Care Med*, 37, 3024–3030.

Kill, C., Leonhardt, A., & Wulf, H. (2003). Lactic acidosis after short-term infusion of propofol for anaesthesia in a child with osteogenesis imperfecta. *Paediatr Anaesth*, 13, 823–826.

Koch, M., De Backer, D., & Vincent, J.L. (2004). Lactic acidosis: an early marker of propofol infusion syndrome? *Intensive Care Med*, 30, 522.

Krajcova, A., Waldauf, P., Andel, M., *et al.* (2015). Propofol infusion syndrome: a structured review of experimental studies and 153 published case reports. *Crit Care*, 19, 398.

Mehta, N., DeMunter, C., Habibi, P., *et al.* (1999). Short-term propofol infusions in children. *Lancet*, 354, 866–867.

Parke, T.J., Stevens, J.E., Rice, A.S., *et al.* (1992). Metabolic acidosis and fatal myocardial failure after propofol infusion in children: five case reports. *BMJ*, 305, 613–616.

Vanlander, A.V., Okun, J.G., de Jaeger, A., *et al.* (2015). Possible pathogenic mechanism of propofol infusion syndrome involves coenzyme Q. *Anesthesiology*, 122, 343–352.

Vasile, B., Rasulo, F., Candiani, A., *et al.* (2003). The pathophysiology of propofol infusion syndrome: a simple name for a complex syndrome. *Intensive Care Med*, 29, 1417–1425.

Wolf, A., Weir, P., Segar, P., *et al.* (2001). Impaired fatty acid oxidation in propofol infusion syndrome. *Lancet*, 357, 606–607.

6.6 Systemic Effect of Local Treatment

Case

A few decades ago, a 3-month-old girl, weighing 5.3 kg, was scheduled for eye examination and trabeculectomy. Her history included three uneventful general anaesthetics for the extraction of congenital cataracts on both eyes some weeks ago. For 10 days the mother had been administering twice-daily timolol eye drops because of an elevated intraocular pressure. Anaesthesia was induced by mask with nitrous oxide and incremental doses of halothane up to 2.0 V%. At the time of intubation, following 1.5 mg atracurium, a heart rate of 80 beats per minute rapidly dropping to 60, a greyish appearance and a blood pressure of 45/20 mmHg alarmed the anaesthetist.

Halothane was immediately turned down to 0.2 V%, and 0.1 mg of atropine and a fluid bolus of 40 ml (8 ml/kg) of Ringer's lactate were administered. The heart rate increased to 170 and the blood pressure gradually returned to normal values. The further course of the anaesthetic was uneventful.

Discussion

This case of an exaggerated reaction to a carefully performed halothane induction with profound bradycardia and hypotension illustrates the possible **systemic effects** of locally administered **eye drops**, in this case the beta-blocker timolol. This is especially a problem in small children, in whom, compared to adults, a similar amount of drug has to be given locally in order to achieve the necessary intraocular target concentration; it is estimated that a newborn requires 50% of the adult dosage and a 6-year-old child 90%. However, the absorbing surfaces are similar, but the absorbed amount is distributed to a much smaller volume of distribution (Farkouh *et al.* 2016). After the administration of timolol eye drops more than 10 times higher plasma concentrations were observed in young infants compared to adults (Passo *et al.* 1984). Systemic absorption is especially effective when the compound comes into contact with the nasal mucosa. During general anaesthesia, diminished tear production and the absence of eyelid movements will reduce the absorption, but general anaesthesia also impairs the reactivity of the autonomic nervous system to maintain cardiovascular stability.

Timolol, a beta-blocker, can lead to hypotension and bradycardia even when locally applied (Maenpaa & Pelkonen 2016). In addition it is metabolized by CYP2D6 and the metabolic rate underlies pharmacogenetic differences; especially high concentrations are found in poor metabolizers. Bradycardia and hypotension during anaesthesia has been reported in adults (Mishra *et al.* 1983), and it can occur in children too, as this case shows.

Phenylephrine is widely used in ophthalmic and ENT surgery in order to provide mydriasis and a bloodless field. Systemically absorbed, it causes vasoconstriction, hypertension, reflex bradycardia and cardiac failure (Baldwin & Morley 2002, Sbaraglia *et al.* 2014). The 10% solution was never popular for paediatric use and is dangerous (Abdelhalim *et al.* 2012); but the 2.5% solution can also cause severe side effects (Ahmed *et al.* 2009, Baldwin & Morley 2002). Therefore, a combination of even more diluted phenylephrine combined with tropicamide (an anticholinergic agent) is used by some practitioners for eye examinations in preterm babies. Following nasal administration of 0.1 ml/kg of a 0.25% or 0.5% solution of phenylephrine, the peak plasma concentration was achieved after 14 minutes and only a moderate increase of blood pressure was observed in children (Christensen *et al.* 2017).

Another situation is the occurrence of an **unexplained mydriasis** or anisocoria in patients in whom drugs intended for another use have accidentally come into direct contact with the eye. In the context of anaesthesia and trauma (cf. Case 5.3), the anaesthetist may immediately assume an intracranial pathology. But an accidental splash of an alpha-1-adrenergic or vagolytic compound into the eye can cause profound mydriasis too (Schmidt *et al.* 2006). The author remembers a child going for an emergency CT scan simply because the nasal drops intended for nasal decongestion had splashed into the eye; in another situation, an anaesthesia nurse developed mydriasis when she rubbed her eyes after drawing up a syringe containing atropine. Often, in such cases, forensic methods have to be used to find out the origin.

Summary and Recommendations

This case shows that topically applied drugs get absorbed and can lead to severe side effects.

Potent medications require careful dosing; it is important to respect the dosing interval and to wait some minutes until a sufficient mydriasis has developed.

Remember that an unexplained mydriasis could be caused by an accidental splash of an alpha-agonist or an anticholinergic compound.

References

Abdelhalim, A.A., Mostafa, M., Abdulmomen, A., *et al.* (2012). Severe hypertension and pulmonary edema associated with systemic absorption of topical phenylephrine in a child during retinal surgery. *Saudi J Anaesth*, 6, 285–288.

Ahmed, N., Riad, W., Altorpaq, A., *et al.* (2009). Ocular phenylephrine 2.5% continues to be dangerous. *BMJ Case Rep*, 2009, pii: bcr08.2008.0795.

Baldwin, F.J. & Morley, A.P. (2002). Intraoperative pulmonary oedema in a child following systemic absorption of phenylephrine eyedrops. *Br J Anaesth*, 88, 440–442.

Christensen, L.K., Armstead, V.E., Bilyeu, D.P., *et al.* (2017). Hemodynamic responses and plasma phenylephrine concentrations associated with intranasal phenylephrine in children. *Paediatr Anaesth*, 27, 768–773.

Farkouh, A., Frigo, P., & Czejka, M. (2016). Systemic side effects of eye drops: a pharmacokinetic perspective. *Clin Ophthalmol*, 10, 2433–2441.

Maenpaa, J. & Pelkonen, O. (2016). Cardiac safety of ophthalmic timolol. *Expert Opin Drug Saf*, 15, 1549–1561.

Mishra, P., Calvey, T.N., Williams, N.E., *et al.* (1983). Intraoperative bradycardia and hypotension associated with timolol and pilocarpine eye drops. *Br J Anaesth*, 55, 897–899.

Passo, M.S., Palmer, E.A., & Van Buskirk, E.M. (1984). Plasma timolol in glaucoma patients. *Ophthalmology*, 91, 1361–1363.

Sbaraglia, F., Mores, N., Garra, R., *et al.* (2014). Phenylephrine eye drops in pediatric patients undergoing ophthalmic surgery: incidence, presentation, and management of complications during general anesthesia. *Paediatr Anaesth*, 24, 400–405.

Schmidt, J., Irouschek, A., & Hemmerling, T.M. (2006). Unilateral mydriasis after anesthesia from nasal atropine administration. *Paediatr Anaesth*, 16, 362–363.

Case

Several decades ago, a 2 6/12-year-old girl, weighing 12 kg, had been operated on because of perforated appendicitis. Intraoperatively, 'paediatric solution' containing 5% glucose and 50 mmol/l sodium was given at a maintenance rate, and in addition Ringer's lactate to achieve haemodynamic stability and replace the gastrointestinal losses. Before surgery she was alternately crying and wanting her mother. In the late evening, after emergence from anaesthesia, the child was extubated and transferred to the corridor on the ward. Because of persistent vomiting the infusion rate of the paediatric maintenance infusion was increased. After midnight, nurses found her unarousable, lying in the vomit and breathing inadequately. Aspiration was considered to be the main problem. The patient was transferred in a hurry to the local intensive care unit; she was obviously cyanotic (this case occurred before pulse oximetry was available) and was intubated orally by the anaesthetist, and the cyanotic appearance vanished.

The oral tube was exchanged for a nasal one, and transfer by ambulance to the paediatric hospital was organized. During transport one pupil was noted to be larger than the other, and at the time of arrival both pupils were maximally dilated and unreactive to light. The plasma sodium concentration was found to be far below normal. Despite maximal treatment the patient was declared brain-dead. The post-mortem examination revealed a massive brain oedema, but also a moderately sized tumour in the cerebellar region.

Discussion

This case illustrates all the elements of a catastrophic course towards lethal brain oedema caused by **hyponatraemia**: a small child, fever and illness, administration of a hypotonic infusion solution, insufficient laboratory tests, and finally a concomitant cerebral pathology. This cerebellar tumour was completely asymptomatic before the acute illness, so it is likely that the hyponatraemia was the main driving force for the development of massive brain oedema.

This story happened a long time ago, and for that time the child received the **standard of care.** Today the child would have been transferred for treatment to a paediatric centre and monitored. Pulse oximetry would now be available, and the measurement of sodium would be easy. But, most important, hypotonic fluids would not have been used in perioperative paediatric medicine (Sümpelmann *et al.* 2017).

The **stress reaction**, trauma, illness, surgery and anaesthesia, triggers antidiuretic hormone secretion in order to preserve the stores of water in the body. The administration of free water by oral intake or infusion therapy leads to hyponatraemia, brain oedema and at worst death. One solution would be to restrict the amount of water given; however, this approach is difficult to manage and will result in a low urine output. A more convenient approach is to administer a solution with high sodium content, accepting moderate weight gain but at the same time reducing the risk of life-threatening hyponatraemia. Historically, the 'paediatric' hyponatraemic solutions and dosing formulas were initiated by Holliday and Segar based on energy expenditure and maximum obtainable concentrated urine (Steurer & Berger 2011). These hypotonic solutions, based on these assumptions, were widely used in paediatric practice and led to an epidemic of **iatrogenic hyponatraemia** (Arieff *et al.* 1992, Moritz & Ayus 2003, Pfenninger 1992). In the United States, in the 1980s, up to 600 children died annually because of an inadequate infusion regime (Arieff *et al.* 1992). Especially in the first half of his professional career, the author saw various cases of severe hyponatraemia including two deaths caused by an inadequate perioperative infusion therapy. Both children probably would not have died if adequate fluid therapy – or none – had been provided. It has to be noted that fatal hyponatraemia can develop very rapidly, within less than 24 hours, e.g. in a child with tonsillectomy, protracted vomiting and the infusion of free water (Sicot & Laxenaire 2007).

Today it is strongly recommended to use isotonic solutions with high sodium content and to **ban hypotonic solutions** in the field of acute paediatric medicine (Moritz & Ayus 2003). Normal saline was traditionally used in the United States (Moritz & Ayus 2003); however, a **balanced salt solution** containing metabolizable anions, such as lactate, malate or acetate, is preferable because it maintains acid–base balance and avoids hyperchloraemic acidosis (Table 6.7; cf. Case 6.8). The use of isotonic solutions is clearly advantageous outside of anaesthesia and surgery too, as shown in randomized controlled trials (Friedman *et al.* 2015) and in meta-analyses (Wang *et al.* 2014).

Despite clear evidence and a relevant mortality related to the use of the old 'paediatric solutions', the anaesthetic community was surprisingly resistant to moving away from this dangerous practice. Even in the second decade of this century hypotonic solutions are still used by some practitioners; the knowledge provided by science is obviously '**lost in translation'**.

The administration of **desmopressin**, e.g. for enhancing coagulation or given daily to children against nocturnal enuresis, exposes these patients to a higher risk of hyponatraemia, and the sodium concentration has to be monitored (Lucchini *et al.* 2013). The **cerebral salt-wasting syndrome**, mainly triggered by various neurosurgical disorders, is characterized by hyponatraemia, dehydration and a high urine sodium loss. The fluid balance is negative in these patients, whereas in **SIADH**, the situation in which concentrations of antidiuretic hormone are inadequate, it tends to be positive.

Table 6.7 The prerequisites of an infusion solution for safe routine paediatric anaesthesia

	Important components	Comments
1.	High sodium concentration	Avoidance of hyponatraemia
2.	Metabolizable anions	Avoidance of hyperchloraemic acidosis
3.	10 mg/ml (1%) glucose	Avoidance of hypoglycaemia

Summary and Recommendations

Iatrogenic hyponatraemia is a threat to sick children. In perioperative settings only isotonic fluids with high sodium content (> 120 mmol/l?) should be used.

The sodium concentration has to be measured in every sick child. Beside infectious parameters, e.g. C-reactive protein (CRP), the sodium concentration is the single most important laboratory parameter in emergency paediatric medicine. It is often an index of the severity of the disease.

The long persistence of inadequate infusion regimes in paediatric anaesthesia is an impressive illustration of the fact that it often takes decades until scientific knowledge is transferred into clinical practice; it is 'lost in translation'.

References

Arieff, A.I., Ayus, J.C., & Fraser, C.L. (1992). Hyponatraemia and death or permanent brain damage in healthy children. *BMJ*, 304, 1218–1222.

Friedman, J.N., Beck, C.E., DeGroot, J., *et al.* (2015). Comparison of isotonic and hypotonic intravenous maintenance fluids: a randomized clinical trial. *JAMA Pediatr*, 169, 445–451.

Lucchini, B., Simonetti, G.D., Ceschi, A., *et al.* (2013). Severe signs of hyponatremia secondary to desmopressin treatment for enuresis: a systematic review. *J Pediatr Urol*, 9, 1049–1053.

Moritz, M.L. & Ayus, J.C. (2003). Prevention of hospital-acquired hyponatremia: a case for using isotonic saline. *Pediatrics*, 111, 227–230.

Pfenninger, J. (1992). Peri-operative water intoxication: a dangerous and unnecessary complication. *Paediatr Anaesth*, 2, 85–87

Sicot, C. & Laxenaire, M.C. (2007). Death of a child due to posttonsillectomy hyponatraemic encephalopathy [in French]. *Ann Fr Anesth Reanim*, 26, 893–896.

Steurer, M.A. & Berger, T.M. (2011). Infusion therapy for neonates, infants and children [in German]. *Anaesthesist*, 60, 10–22.

Sümpelmann, R., Becke, K., Brenner, S., *et al.* (2017). Perioperative intravenous fluid therapy in children: guidelines from the Association of the Scientific Medical Societies in Germany. *Paediatr Anaesth*, 27, 10–18.

Wang, J., Xu, E., & Xiao, Y. (2014). Isotonic versus hypotonic maintenance IV fluids in hospitalized children: a meta-analysis. *Pediatrics*, 133, 105–113.

Hyperchloraemic Acidosis

Case

Many years ago, a 7 3/12-year-old girl, weighing 25 kg, was scheduled for the resection of a pulmonary cystic echinococcosis in the left lower lobe. Anaesthesia was induced with 5 mg/kg thiopental, 1 μg/kg fentanyl and 0.2 mg/kg mivacurium. Desflurane up to 8 V%, remifentanil 0.1–0.3 μg/kg/min and a continuous infusion of mivacurium were given for maintenance. Caudal morphine 80 μg/kg was given before surgery and intercostal nerve blocks were performed at the end for postoperative pain relief. Dexamethasone 0.3 mg/kg, ranitidine 1 mg/kg and clemastine 0.02 mg/kg were preventively injected in order to attenuate an allergic reaction.

The airway management included a 5F Fogarty balloon catheter inserted through the nostril into the trachea, followed by an orally inserted size 5.0 cuffed endotracheal tube (ETT). Under fibreoptic control the Fogarty catheter was manipulated into the left main-stem bronchus, the necessary volume for occlusion was checked and the catheter was firmly taped in place.

The left lower lobe resection caused diffuse oozing because of multiple adhesions. In addition to Ringer's lactate for maintenance, 500 ml of normal saline and 500 ml of a starch solution (Voluven 130/0.4) were given and cardiovascular stability was maintained. But finally anaemia (haemoglobin 69 g/l) combined with metabolic acidosis at a base excess of −7.6 mmol/l triggered the transfusion of 250 ml of packed red cells. The child was extubated after skin closure; diclofenac, metamizole and minimal doses of a morphine/ketamine mixture by PCA provided good pain relief.

Upon arrival on the PICU, a persisting metabolic acidosis with a base excess of −8.1 mmol/l combined with high sodium and chloride concentrations (146 mmol/l and 121 mmol/l respectively) remained unexplained, until it was realized that this hyperchlor-aemic acidosis was caused in part by the absorption of sodium chloride from the operating field. The theatre nurse had inadvertently provided the surgeon with hypertonic saline 20% (3.4 mmol/ml) for wound irrigation, a solution that was intended for use in case of cyst puncture. The surgeon had realized the mistake because of a whitish film on the instruments, but this was not communicated to the anaesthetic team.

Discussion

This case of unexpected metabolic acidosis during pulmonary resection has been previously reported in part elsewhere (Jöhr *et al.* 2006). It highlights several educational points.

First, **metabolic acidosis** is not a homogeneous entity; it should always prompt further diagnostic reflection. During anaesthesia, acidosis is often considered to be the result of hypoperfusion and lactate accumulation; so it can trigger volume loading and, as in this case, transfusion of red cells. The full diagnostic workup includes the evaluation of lactate, sodium and chloride concentrations (Rehm *et al.* 2004) as well as the calculation of the anion gap. This should be done on a routine basis.

Second, unfortunately, **hyperchloraemic acidosis** is still a very common iatrogenic condition as the result of a traditional infusion regime based on normal saline. The high chloride concentration of 154 mmol/l invariably leads to hyperchloraemic acidosis (cf. Case 6.7). Therefore, suitable solutions for fluid therapy and volume replacement should contain metabolizable anions, such as lactate, acetate or malate (Sümpelmann *et al.* 2017). In this case the intravenous administration of 20 ml/kg of normal saline and 20 ml/kg of a starch solution, which in those days was still diluted in normal saline, had contributed to the development of the hyperchloraemic acidosis. It has to be noted that many drugs, e.g. remifentanil, mivacurium and dopamine, are traditionally diluted with normal saline; especially in neonates, these 'medical fluids' often represent a large part of the totally infused volume during anaesthesia and are responsible for the subsequent hyperchloraemic acidosis. The author's approach was to use a balanced solution for the dilution of drugs; however, the pharmaceutic stability may not be guaranteed by the drug companies. The same thoughts are valid for flushing the arterial line with heparin. In neonatology, hypotonic solutions of sodium acetate are used for umbilical arterial catheters. Only on rare occasions will the intake of chloride via the wound surface be relevant; but 20% sodium chloride contains 20 times more chloride than normal saline, and package of the wound or instillation into a hydatid cyst can lead to massive electrolyte disturbances (Albi *et al.* 2002, Rakic *et al.* 1994). In this case, flushing the pleural cavity with a 20% saline solution certainly contributed to the hyperchloraemic acidosis.

Third, a child with **hydatid disease** is a rare patient for the paediatric anaesthetist living in the Western world. Large tumours can occur in the lung (Dave *et al.* 2004), the liver or other vital organs (Panda *et al.* 2014). The spillage of antigenic material following cyst rupture leading to an anaphylactic reaction is an inherent risk (Marashi *et al.* 2014). Toxic solutions, e.g. 20% saline, alcohol or formalin, are administered into the cysts in order to impede a further spread of the disease (Albi *et al.* 2002, Rakic *et al.* 1994).

Fourth, **lung separation** (Hammer 2004, Letal & Theam 2017) is highly desirable for surgery in a case of pulmonary hydatid disease, because spillage of the cyst contents into the whole bronchial tree can have catastrophic consequences. Double-lumen tubes are considered the gold standard for lung isolation (Letal & Theam 2017); however, they can only be used in children older than 8 years, because the smallest available device is size 26F, which means an outer diameter of 8.7 mm. It was the author's practice always to first check the ability to pass the subglottic region with a cheap well-lubricated ordinary tube with the same outer diameter before preparing the expensive double-lumen tube. Under 8 years of age bronchial blockers are used, e.g. the 5F Arndt bronchial blocker by Cook. It can be passed coaxially as long as the child can be intubated with a size 4.5 ETT, which means approximately 4 years with a cuffed and 1 year with an uncuffed tube. A diameter of at least 4.5 mm is essential to allow free guidance of the 1.7 mm (5F) blocker by the 2.2 mm bronchoscope. Below this age the bronchial blocker has to be inserted in parallel to the ETT. With the coaxial technique the Arndt blocker works well; it contains a nylon wire with a terminal loop at the end which can be used to guide the blocker with the bronchoscope. Once the nylon wire is removed this lumen can be used to deflate or inflate the lung, e.g. by using a Luer lock 50 ml syringe (Fig. 6.8). When using a parallel technique a stiffer blocker with an angulated tip is often advantageous, e.g. a Fogarty catheter. Endobronchial intubation is an option too. Today, a 5F coaxially inserted Arndt blocker would be a very good device for the patient described here.

Finally, this case highlights the importance of **communication** between all members of the team. If the erroneous surgical use of 20% saline had been reported to the anaesthetic team, this knowledge could have led to a more detailed analysis of the metabolic acidosis and perhaps the transfusion would have been avoided. Especially in procedures that are rarely performed, a meticulous briefing is essential, e.g. that 20% saline is for cyst injection and not just replacing normal saline.

Summary and Recommendations

This case highlights that a metabolic acidosis should primarily lead to further diagnostic reflection, and should not trigger reflex-like treatment with volume loading and red cell transfusion.

Iatrogenic hyperchloraemic acidosis is still the most common disturbance of acid–base balance in perioperative medicine. The use of normal saline should be restricted.

Bronchial blockers are an important tool for paediatric lung isolation. The available options have to be known by the practitioner.

This case also illustrates the necessity of continuous communication between all involved caregivers.

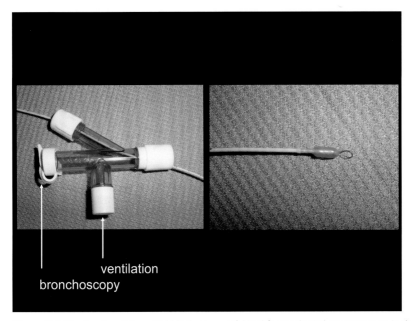

ventilation

bronchoscopy

Figure 6.8 The Arndt endobronchial blocker is a useful tool for paediatric lung separation. In the described case a Fogarty catheter was used, inserted in parallel to the ETT.

References

Albi, A., Baudin, F., Matmar, M., *et al.* (2002). Severe hypernatremia after hypertonic saline irrigation of hydatid cysts. *Anesth Analg*, 95, 1806–1808.

Dave, N., Halbe, A.R., Kadam, P.P., *et al.* (2004). Bilateral pulmonary hydatid cysts in a child: anesthetic management. *Paediatr Anaesth*, 14, 889–890.

Hammer, G.B. (2004). Single-lung ventilation in infants and children. *Paediatr Anaesth*, 14, 98–102.

Jöhr, M., Berger, T.M., & Winiker, H. (2006). Unexpected hypernatremia during pulmonary resection in a 7-year-old child with hydatid disease. *Paediatr Anaesth*, 16, 697–698.

Letal, M. & Theam, M. (2017). Paediatric lung isolation. *BJA Education*, 17, 57–62.

Marashi, S., Hosseini, V.S., Saliminia, A., *et al.* (2014). Anaphylactic shock during pulmonary hydatid cyst surgery. *Anesth Pain Med*, 4, e16725.

Panda, N.B., Batra, Y., Mishra, A., *et al.* (2014). A giant intracranial hydatid cyst in a child: intraoperative anaesthetic concerns. *Indian J Anaesth*, 58, 477–479.

Rakic, M., Vegan, B., Sprung, J., *et al.* (1994). Acute hyperosmolar coma complicating anesthesia for hydatid disease surgery. *Anesthesiology*, 80, 1175–1178.

Rehm, M., Conzen, P.F., Peter, K., *et al.* (2004). The Stewart model. 'Modern' approach to the interpretation of the acid-base metabolism [in German]. *Anaesthesist*, 53, 347–357.

Sümpelmann, R., Becke, K., Brenner, S., *et al.* (2017). Perioperative intravenous fluid therapy in children: guidelines from the Association of the Scientific Medical Societies in Germany. *Paediatr Anaesth*, 27, 10–18.

Case

Several decades ago, close to midnight, a 17-year-old adolescent presented in an emergency department with air hunger and malaise. He was breathing rapidly at large tidal volumes. The attending physician made the presumptive diagnosis of psychogenic hyperventilation and prescribed that the nurse should inject one ampoule of calcium. She was one of the temporary staff and correctly checked back, 'one ampoule of potassium?' showing the vial to the doctor. He, in a hurry and with a rather unfriendly manner, said 'yes this stuff, just inject it now.'

When the nurse started the injection the patient screamed out in pain, and an anaesthetist standing nearby ran to succour; he recognized the coloured label on the vial from afar, screamed 'stop', and attached the leads of the ECG monitor. The tracing showed a loss of sinus rhythm and high T waves as large as the QRS complex. Pain subsided, calcium was injected as scheduled, and the ECG tracing returned to normal.

Discussion

This case of medication error leading to **hyperkalaemia** emphasizes the danger of handling highly concentrated **potassium**. A vial of potassium, e.g. 10 mmol in 10 ml, is the only compound in the armamentarium of the anaesthetist which almost immediately causes cardiac arrest when it is injected directly intravenously. In the 40 years of his medical career the author was aware of three other cases of inadvertent potassium administration, two of them leading to cardiac arrest. In awake patients, the injection into a peripheral vein causes intense pain; this led to early recognition and prevented cardiac arrest in the case described here. When the injection is made through a central venous catheter or during anaesthesia, there is no pain.

Preventive measures are important. In the author's institution, where no paediatric cardiac anaesthesia was performed, there was no absolute need to store potassium in the operating theatre and so this potential source of error could be eliminated by banning this drug from the OR. This case also shows that double-checking medications does not protect from errors when one party does it only pro forma and not driven by the conviction that this communication standard is beneficial.

Apart from iatrogenic errors, the **causes of hyperkalaemia** include the following entities.

First, a too **high potassium load**, too much in too short a time, can induce hyperkalaemia: e.g. rapid transfusion (Smith *et al.* 2008), rhabdomyolysis, tumour lysis syndrome (Osthaus *et al.* 2008) or transfusion reaction. The **rapid transfusion** of red blood cells brings a potassium load which cannot be acutely handled by the organism, induces hyperkalaemia and is a major cause of paediatric cardiac arrest (Bhananker *et al.* 2007). The population at risk are mainly neonates and infants receiving a replacement of one blood volume or more (Lee *et al.* 2014). A rapid transfusion is often needed in the presence of previously underestimated blood loss, and therefore it is often combined with hypotension and acidosis. Prolonged storage of red cells as well as irradiated blood products, especially when transfused through very narrow lines under high pressure, are additional risk factors; but storage time is the most important of these (Miller & Schlueter 2004). If a massive transfusion is anticipated, washing of banked blood products can reduce the amount of potassium which would be otherwise co-administered with the red blood cells (Gruber *et al.* 2013). The author remembers a severely injured toddler, after a fall from the fourth floor, who ultimately died on the table during massive transfusion because of a liver laceration and multiple fractures. Retrospectively, although acutely not measured, hyperkalaemia was the most likely acute cause of cardiac arrest.

Second, a **potassium shift** from intracellular to extracellular space in the presence of acidosis occurs rapidly. When the potassium level is already high, often a **minimal additional change** is sufficient to induce life-threatening symptoms. The author remembers a 15-year-old intoxicated girl who was found outdoors after lying there for several hours. In the hospital, the injection of naloxone made her very agitated; she only calmed down after repeated doses of diazepam, but then she arrested. Resuscitation was unsuccessful for more than 15 minutes despite repeated doses of adrenaline and a trial of defibrillation. It was only when calcium was injected, as a desperate last resort, that the heart returned to sinus rhythm. And only now was a high potassium concentration discovered, and hours later the myonecrosis at the buttocks and the legs became apparent. Diazepam-induced hypoventilation and respiratory acidosis had been sufficient to increase the potassium concentration further and to induce cardiac arrest.

Third, **insufficient elimination** can be caused by renal failure, medications or hormonal factors. Insufficient cortisol concentrations, e.g. in inefficiently substituted children with congenital adrenal hyperplasia, typically cause hyperkalaemia (Ruppen *et al.* 2003).

For an early **diagnosis** a high index of suspicion is needed; e.g. in severely injured patients the potassium concentration should be checked as soon as the patient arrives in the emergency room. Normally, it is well below normal, because the high catecholamine concentrations cause a potassium shift into the cells. A normal potassium concentration under such circumstances makes one suspicious for an underlying condition, e.g. an ongoing rhabdomyolysis or a pre-existing renal insufficiency.

The key to successful **treatment** is early recognition (Masilamani & van der Voort 2012). Perioperatively, when the first signs are visible, e.g. a T-wave elevation in the ECG tracing, calcium should be injected immediately before laboratory results are available and one should not wait for cardiac arrest. Only then is further treatment planned (Table 6.9). Insulin together with glucose causes a shift of potassium from the extracellular to the intracellular space; the basic rule to be remembered is: 1 U insulin + 3–5 grams of glucose shift 1 mmol potassium from the extracellular to the intracellular space. In the non-diabetic child, a glucose-containing infusion on its own will initiate a decline in the potassium concentration. If a fixed mixture of glucose and insulin (e.g. 5:1) is used, rapid administration will usually cause hyperglycaemia, and slow administration a decline in the glucose concentration; in either case, the glucose concentration has to be monitored. Of course, every ongoing potassium administration should be stopped.

Table 6.9 The principles of treating hyperkalaemia

Mechanism	Compound	Dose	Comments
Reduced toxicity	Calcium	20 mg/kg $CaCl_2$ or 60 mg/kg Ca gluconate	Immediate action, repeatedly if needed
Intracellular shift	Sodium bicarbonate	1–2 mmol/kg	Even in the absence of acidosis
	Insulin + glucose	0.1 U/kg insulin + 0.5 g/kg glucose over 30 minutes	Followed by a separate infusion of 0.5 g/kg/h (5–8 mg/kg/min) glucose and 0.05 U/kg/h insulin
	β-agonists, e.g. salbutamol	By inhalation or 4 μg/kg over 5 min i.v.	Rapid onset of action; in case of hypotension consider a low-dose adrenaline infusion
Elimination	Diuretics and fluids	Furosemide 0.5–1 mg/kg	
	Calcium resonium	1 g/kg oral or rectal	Slow onset of action
	Dialysis Haemofiltration		In case of renal failure

Summary and Recommendations

This story of iatrogenic hyperkalaemia illustrates the importance of a strict communication discipline in medicine; but even closed-loop communication does not work if one partner is not listening.

Hyperkalaemia is a treatable condition, and it is of paramount importance to think of it. In every unsuccessful resuscitation you should have recourse to calcium, especially when the history leading to cardiac arrest is unknown.

A rapid transfusion of red blood cells to neonates and infants is a situation at high risk; any suspicion of an elevated T wave should trigger the injection of calcium.

References

Bhananker, S.M., Ramamoorthy, C., Geiduschek, J.M., et al. (2007). Anesthesia-related cardiac arrest in children: update from the Pediatric Perioperative Cardiac Arrest Registry. *Anesth Analg*, 105, 344–350.

Gruber, M., Breu, A., Frauendorf, M., et al. (2013). Washing of banked blood by three different blood salvage devices. *Transfusion*, 53, 1001–1009.

Lee, A.C., Reduque, L.L., Luban, N.L., et al. (2014). Transfusion-associated hyperkalemic cardiac arrest in pediatric patients receiving massive transfusion. *Transfusion*, 54, 244–254.

Masilamani, K. & van der Voort, J. (2012). The management of acute hyperkalaemia in neonates and children. *Arch Dis Child*, 97, 376–380.

Miller, M.A. & Schlueter, A.J. (2004). Transfusions via hand-held syringes and small-gauge needles as risk factors for hyperkalemia. *Transfusion*, 44, 373–381.

Osthaus, W.A., Linderkamp, C., Bunte, C., et al. (2008). Tumor lysis associated with dexamethasone use in a child with leukemia. *Paediatr Anaesth*, 18, 268–270.

Ruppen, W., Hagenbuch, N., Jöhr, M., *et al.* (2003). Cardiac arrest in an infant with congenital adrenal hyperplasia.

Acta Anaesthesiol Scand, 47, 104–105.

Smith, H.M., Farrow, S.J., Ackerman, J.D., *et al.* (2008). Cardiac arrests associated with hyperkalemia during red blood cell transfusion: a case series. *Anesth Analg*, 106, 1062–1069.

Prolonged Paralysis

Case

Many years ago, a 1 3/12-year-old girl, 10 kg, was brought to theatre for urgent repair of a large skin laceration. She had received rectal midazolam for premedication and EMLA cream had been applied. Venous access was achieved and anaesthesia induced by injecting thiopental 7.5 mg/kg and mivacurium 0.2 mg/kg. A size 3.5 cuffed endotracheal tube was inserted under optimal conditions and anaesthesia was maintained with sevoflurane.

At the end of the surgical procedure, 70 minutes after induction, muscle response was absent following train-of-four (TOF) stimulation and the post-tetanic count was zero. This constellation was interpreted as indicating the presence of an atypical cholinesterase. After a brief discussion with the team, the decision was made to keep the child in the holding area of the operating block. The patient was transferred to her bed, still intubated and kept asleep with sevoflurane. The parents were called, and they sat beside their peacefully sleeping daughter while the anaesthetist explained that everything was fine and there was no complication, but that an unexpected inherited trait meant that their daughter dealt with one of the anaesthetic compounds in a different way.

Later, 2½ hours after the injection of mivacurium, the first twitch could be felt after post-tetanic-count stimulation, and when three twitches were countable neostigmine 50 µg/kg and glycopyrrolate 10 µg/kg were injected. Soon afterwards, the first twitch appeared after TOF stimulation, but further recovery was rather slow. It was not until 30 minutes after reversal, 3¼ hours after mivacurium, that neuromuscular function was fully recovered with no fading after double-burst stimulation (Fig. 6.10). The patient was extubated and transferred to the ward. A medical emergency card was given to the parents stating 'prolonged action (> 3 hours) of mivacurium'.

Discussion

In general, **prolonged paralysis** can be caused by altered metabolism, overdose or altered pharmacodynamics.

This case illustrates **altered metabolism**; it shows a typical time course of prolonged paralysis after mivacurium caused by a **butyrylcholinesterase** (BChE, formerly known as pseudocholinesterase) variant (Lejus *et al.* 1998). BChE hydrolyses mivacurium and succinylcholine. Patients with mutations in the BChE gene will hydrolyse these compounds to a lesser extent and are at risk for a prolonged paralysis. Whereas at the beginning of this century the distinction was mainly between wild-type and atypical variant, with heterozygote patients experiencing moderate prolongation of the blockade and homozygotes a prolongation for 2–12 hours (Cerf *et al.* 2002), today the situation looks much more

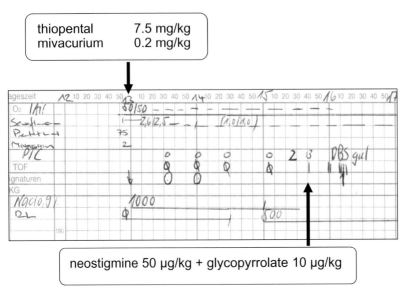

Figure 6.10 The time course of paralysis in the described patient

complex because an increasing number of mutations are described at the BChE gene, with a range of clinical significance (Wichmann *et al.* 2016). In daily clinical practice, a patient homozygote for the atypical variant will be a rare event (1:2500) for the individual anaesthetist, but heterozygote patients with some prolongation of the blockade may be as common as 20% (Bretlau *et al.* 2013).

Clinically, **diagnostics** are based on neuromuscular monitoring. This allows the timely diagnosis of a prolonged action (Cassel *et al.* 2014). It is of paramount importance not to re-dose or to run an infusion of mivacurium in a patient with disturbed metabolism. In normal patients a relevant part of mivacurium is destroyed by BChE before it reaches the neuromuscular junction; in case of an atypical variant, however, much higher concentrations reach the neuromuscular junction, and, similar to an overdose, a very rapid onset results. Therefore, looking at the rate of disappearance of the twitches during induction allows some prognosis about the duration of the blockade in the individual patient. Biochemically, in patients with variants, the activity of BChE is usually reduced, but more important it is qualitatively different and reacts in a different way to inhibitors, such as fluoride and dibucaine. The normal BChE is inhibited to a large extent by dibucaine, the homozygote atypical variant by less than 30%. For scientific research, molecular biology can identify the individual mutations. In clinical reality, biochemical examinations are not essential; it is important that the patient knows that the action of mivacurium and succinylcholine will be prolonged, and that other members of the family may be affected too.

The **treatment** consists in early recognition, and then continued sedation and ventilation until some spontaneous recovery occurs, at which point reversal with neostigmine can be planned. Injected cholinesterase accelerates the breakdown of mivacurium, but it is neither universally available nor a generally recommended practice (Ostergaard *et al.* 2005). Homozygote patients are rare and occur at a rate of 1:2500; nevertheless, every institution should have a plan of how to deal with such a situation. Transfer to a paediatric intensive care unit (PICU) is an option, but parents are alarmed and ventilation is often prolonged, because PICU staff may be less familiar with neuromuscular monitoring and reversal. Taking care of the patient and the family in the holding area may be an optimal solution. **Communication** to parents is crucial; they have to know that this altered metabolism is just a variation of nature, like different hair colours, and has no impact on the normal life of their child; in fact the patient's enzyme is even 'stronger', as it is not blocked by dibucaine. For a small single-handed outpatient unit such a patient blocking a whole busy surgical list may be a problem; this was for several practitioners the reason for abandoning the use of mivacurium.

In case of prolonged paralysis after **succinylcholine** the course of action is identical. With a homozygote atypical variant the signs of a non-depolarizing block, a phase II block (Jurkolow *et al.* 2014), become apparent and reversal with neostigmine can be successfully used.

Prolonged paralysis can be the consequence of **overdose**. The author remembers an infant who received 2 mg/kg mivacurium over a few minutes, because an error by a factor of 10 in running a mivacurium infusion occurred which was discovered after a delay of 6 minutes. Nonetheless, recovery started during the case and was, once it had begun, as rapid as normal. The elimination of the steroid compounds rocuronium, vecuronium and pancuronium is dependent on liver and kidney function. The author remembers a 1-year-old child with cardiomyopathy and multiorgan failure who, based on clinical judgement, received seven doses of 0.1 mg/kg pancuronium over the first 36 hours on the PICU. It was not until 49 hours after the last dose of pancuronium that a post-tetanic count of two could be measured, and the first spontaneous movements were observed after 67 hours. Increased sensitivity, **altered pharmacodynamics**, typically occur with some neuromuscular diseases, e.g. myasthenia gravis (cf. Case 7.2).

BChE is also responsible for metabolism of chloroprocaine. In contrast, esmolol and remifentanil breakdown are not BChE-dependent; they are metabolized by other non-specific esterases. Chloroprocaine has seen some revival in paediatric anaesthesia and toxicity has been described after the paediatric use of the compound, but in none of the cases was it related to altered metabolism (Veneziano & Tobias 2017).

Summary and Recommendations

Neuromuscular monitoring is the key to the safe administration of neuromuscular blocking agents. It allows correct dosing, the assurance of full recovery and the detection of abnormalities.

The variability of butyrylcholinesterase is a typical example of the impact of pharmacogenetics on clinical practice.

Neuromuscular blocking agents, which are dependent on liver and kidney for elimination, should be carefully dosed in the presence of organ dysfunction.

References

Bretlau, C., Sorensen, M.K., Vedersoe, A.L., et al. (2013). Response to succinylcholine in patients carrying the K-variant of the butyrylcholinesterase gene. *Anesth Analg*, 116, 596–601.

Cassel, J., Staehr-Rye, A.K., Nielsen, C.V., et al. (2014). Use of neuromuscular monitoring to detect prolonged effect of succinylcholine or mivacurium: three case reports. *Acta Anaesthesiol Scand*, 58, 1040–1043.

Cerf, C., Mesguish, M., Gabriel, I., *et al.* (2002). Screening patients with prolonged neuromuscular blockade after succinylcholine and mivacurium. *Anesth Analg*, 94, 461–466.

Jurkolow, G., Fuchs-Buder, T., Lemoine, A., *et al.* (2014). Prolonged phase II neuromuscular blockade following succinylcholine administration [in French]. *Ann Fr Anesth Reanim*, 33, 176–177.

Lejus, C., Blanloeil, Y., Le, R.N., *et al.* (1998). Prolonged mivacurium neuromuscular block in children. *Paediatr Anaesth*, 8, 433–435.

Ostergaard, D., Viby-Mogensen, J., Rasmussen, S.N., *et al.* (2005). Pharmacokinetics and pharmacodynamics of mivacurium in patients phenotypically homozygous for the atypical plasma cholinesterase variant: effect of injection of human cholinesterase. *Anesthesiology*, 102, 1124–1132.

Veneziano, G. & Tobias, J.D. (2017). Chloroprocaine for epidural anesthesia in infants and children. *Paediatr Anaesth*, 27, 581–590.

Wichmann, S., Faerk, G., Bundgaard, J.R., *et al.* (2016). Patients with prolonged effect of succinylcholine or mivacurium had novel mutations in the butyrylcholinesterase gene. *Pharmacogenet Genomics*, 26, 351–356.

Case

Many years ago, a 15-year-old boy, 61 kg, was scheduled for bat ear surgery. After oral premedication with 15 mg midazolam, anaesthesia was induced with 150 µg (2.5 µg/kg) fentanyl and propofol by target-controlled infusion (TCI) using the Paedfusor protocol. After the administration of 40 mg (0.7 mg/kg) rocuronium the airway was secured with a cuffed size 7.0 preformed endotracheal tube. Paracetamol and metamizole were given for additional postoperative analgesia, dexamethasone 8 mg and ondansetron 4 mg for prevention of postoperative vomiting (Fig. 6.11). In addition the site of surgical incision was infiltrated with bupivacaine 0.25% with adrenaline.

Over the duration of 140 minutes propofol was dosed at a plasma target concentration between 3 and 6 µg/ml with the aim of maintaining the BIS in the range 20–30. Propofol was stopped 10 minutes before skin closure, and at the time of the removal of the BIS electrode for the application of the bandage the last reading was 26. Over the procedure, a total dose of 250 µg fentanyl had been given.

With a delay of 5 minutes the patient breathed spontaneously; but over 90 minutes there was only a weak cough reflex, no reaction to painful stimuli and a bilateral mydriasis with pupils reacting to light. Flumazenil 10 µg/kg and naloxone 2 µg/kg showed no effect; but physostigmine 40 µg/kg given slowly over 10 minutes led immediately to an arousal reaction. A central anticholinergic syndrome was presumptively diagnosed.

Discussion

This case of **delayed awakening** can be easily explained by an **overdose** of propofol in a sensitive patient. A BIS target of 20–30 was certainly too low, and too much propofol was given. Using the TIVA-Trainer (software for simulating pharmacokinetics which runs on a personal computer) with the Paedfusor protocol the plasma concentrations were simulated to be < 2.0 µg/ml, < 1.5 µg/ml and < 1.0 µg/ml at 30, 50 and 80 minutes respectively. Awakening can be expected at around 1.5 µg/ml. Therefore, even for an average patient, a delay to awakening of around 1 hour could have been expected and, in addition, large interindividual differences exist. Propofol has to be dosed according to clinical need, and the use of a TCI pump alone does not protect against an overdose. Up to 12 years of age the Paedfusor (Marsh *et al.* 1991) pharmacokinetics, in a linear fashion with exception of the clearance, takes only body weight into account (Absalom & Kenny 2005), whereas the Schnider protocol is much more sophisticated. It describes the reality better and may be the preferred protocol for TCI in children above 6 years of age (Rigouzzo *et al.* 2010). Opioids have a propofol-sparing effect and allow a reduction in the amount of propofol. This is

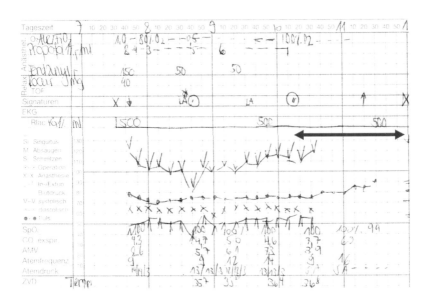

Figure 6.11 The anaesthesia chart of this patient with unexpected slow recovery

beneficial because propofol has a rapid increase of context-sensitive half-life in children (McFarlan *et al.* 1999). Therefore, this case also shows that fentanyl may not be the optimal opioid for a TIVA in children. Remifentanil, with its rapid elimination, can be given in a much higher dose without a clinically relevant prolonged recovery time.

Delayed awakening should always prompt a vigorous evaluation of **differential diagnoses**, which should include among others residual drug action, intracranial pathology, epilepsy, intoxication, hypoglycaemia, hyponatraemia, hypercalcaemia, hypoxaemia, hypercapnia, hypothermia and finally central anticholinergic syndrome. Blood gases, glucose and electrolytes can easily be checked today by point-of-care measurements, whereas a postictal state or intoxication is more difficult to exclude in the busy perioperative environment. In case of trauma or after neurosurgery, early imaging has to be considered, to exclude an intracranial bleed.

Central anticholinergic syndrome (CAS) is characterized by an absolute or relative deficiency of acetylcholine, an essential neurotransmitter in the central nervous system (CNS). It is typically caused by an overdose of anticholinergic agents, which easily cross the blood–brain barrier, e.g. atropine, scopolamine or biperiden (Kulka *et al.* 2004, Schultz *et al.* 2002). Since the beginning of this century, or earlier, most practitioners no longer administer anticholinergic agents on a routine basis (Jöhr 1999); however, CAS is still being diagnosed, as many other compounds have been incriminated too, e.g. opioids, propofol, benzodiazepines, ketamine, halogenated agents or even local anaesthetics. It has to be noted that although the exact mechanism of anaesthesia is surprisingly still unknown, an interaction with cholinergic transmission has been postulated (Kopp Lugli *et al.* 2009). The administration of physostigmine, a cholinesterase inhibitor which crosses the blood–brain barrier, can reverse hypnosis induced by sevoflurane, ketamine or propofol (Meuret *et al.*

Table 6.11 The presence of at least one central and two peripheral signs raises the suspicion of a central anticholinergic syndrome (CAS)

Central signs	Peripheral signs
Sedation, coma	Mydriasis
Excitation	Dry mouth
Disorientation	Tachycardia, dysrhythmia
Hyperpyrexia	Flush
Convulsion	Impaired micturition

2000). Therefore, in this case, the effectiveness of physostigmine could have been a non-specific effect and does not necessarily prove an underlying CAS.

According to current teaching, the presence of one central and two peripheral symptoms raises the suspicion of CAS (Table 6.11); the **diagnosis** is confirmed by the disappearance of the symptoms following the administration of physostigmine.

In many patients some of these symptoms may be seen over the course of a general anaesthetic, especially during emergence. Therefore, the author doubts the existence of a clear CAS entity, and he is convinced that, except for an anticholinergic overdose, CAS is mostly used as a non-specific catch-all for a variety of poorly understood conditions which have in common only that they react to physostigmine. However, the author remembers a preschool child who definitively suffered from CAS: he had received an overdose of metoclopramide, two ampoules, in a non-paediatric hospital, which induced the typical extrapyramidal side effects. Therefore, biperiden was indicated, but unfortunately because of an error in calculating the dose a 10-fold overdose was given (Doherty & McDonnell 2012). This resulted in coma, and physostigmine 30 μg/kg/h had to be infused over several days. Physostigmine has a short half-life of 20–30 minutes. Therefore, not infrequently, repeated dosing or an infusion is needed.

Summary and Recommendations

Anaesthetic overdose is a common cause of delayed awakening. The art of correct dosing takes different factors into account: clinical signs and EEG-based parameters as well as the selection of the optimal drugs.

Central anticholinergic syndrome (CAS) is typically caused by too high a dose of an anticholinergic agent; in addition, in the author's experience, the term is often used to give a name to unexplained clinical situations with delayed awakening and a positive reaction to physostigmine.

Delayed awakening should initiate an investigation to exclude common causes such as glucose, sodium, blood gas and CNS pathology.

References

Absalom, A. & Kenny, G. (2005). 'Paedfusor' pharmacokinetic data set. Br J Anaesth, 95, 110.

Doherty, C. & McDonnell, C. (2012). Tenfold medication errors: 5 years' experience at a university-affiliated pediatric hospital. Pediatrics, 129, 916–924.

Jöhr, M. (1999). Is it time to question the routine use of anticholinergic agents in paediatric anaesthesia? *Paediatr Anaesth*, 9, 99–101.

Kopp Lugli, A., Yost, C.S., & Kindler, C.H. (2009). Anaesthetic mechanisms: update on the challenge of unravelling the mystery of anaesthesia. *Eur J Anaesthesiol*, 26, 807–820.

Kulka, P.J., Toker, H., Heim, J., *et al.* (2004). Suspected central anticholinergic syndrome in a 6-week-old infant. *Anesth Analg*, 99, 1376–1378.

Marsh, B., White, M., Morton, N., *et al.* (1991). Pharmacokinetic model driven infusion of propofol in children. *Br J Anaesth*, 67, 41–48.

McFarlan, C.S., Anderson, B.J., & Short, T.G. (1999). The use of propofol infusions in paediatric anaesthesia: a practical guide. *Paediatr Anaesth*, 9, 209–216.

Meuret, P., Backman, S.B., Bonhomme, V., *et al.* (2000). Physostigmine reverses propofol-induced unconsciousness and attenuation of the auditory steady state response and bispectral index in human volunteers. *Anesthesiology*, 93, 708–717.

Rigouzzo, A., Servin, F., & Constant, I. (2010). Pharmacokinetic-pharmacodynamic modeling of propofol in children. *Anesthesiology*, 113, 343–352.

Schultz, U., Idelberger, R., Rossaint, R., *et al.* (2002). Central anticholinergic syndrome in a child undergoing circumcision. *Acta Anaesthesiol Scand*, 46, 224–226.

Emergence Delirium

Case

More than two decades ago, a 10-month-old boy, 9 kg, was scheduled for meatoplasty and circumcision in the presence of distal glandular hypospadias. After rectal premedication with 9 mg midazolam an uneventful induction of anaesthesia was performed using the new agent sevoflurane. The airway was secured with a classic type laryngeal mask airway (LMA) size 1.5. A caudal block as well as a penile block were performed and 12.5 mg rectal diclofenac was administered for postoperative analgesia. The child breathed spontaneously over the 60-minute procedure with perfectly working regional blocks. The LMA was removed when the child showed spontaneous movements. A few minutes later, the venous access was taken out and the peacefully sleeping child was transferred to the day surgery unit.

Forty minutes later, the nurse called the anaesthetist because the child was inconsolable and thrashing around. All efforts by the parents to calm him down, as well as a dose of rectal paracetamol, had had no effect at all. The anaesthetist decided to give an additional dose of midazolam, but it was only after 30 minutes that the child became quiet and fell into a deep sleep. Two hours later the boy woke up, drank his normal ration of formula milk, showed normal behaviour and seemed to be comfortable and pain-free. He was discharged home shortly afterwards.

Discussion

This case shows a typical **emergence delirium** in an apparently pain-free child. The introduction of the newer agents sevoflurane and desflurane enabled rapid recovery and brought the problem of postoperative agitation to the surface (Jöhr 2002). But it was not until 1997 that it became clear that agitation was much more prominent than it had been in the era of halothane (Aono *et al.* 1997). Whereas initially the phenomenon was attributed to rapid recovery and insufficiently treated pain, it rapidly became clear that agitation can occur unrelated to pain, even after anaesthesia and no surgery (Cravero *et al.* 2000); it seems to be a specific drug effect. Often these children present with the signs of delirium with a fluctuating mental state and unawareness of the surroundings. A commonly used scoring system was presented by Sikich and Lerman (2004). Pain, of course, has always to be ruled out in an agitated child (Somaini *et al.* 2015), and inconsolable crying and thrashing around can be caused by pain as well as delirium. The three predominant findings supporting the **diagnosis** of a delirium are: absence of eye contact with caregivers, absence of purposeful movements, and unawareness of surroundings.

The **pathophysiology** is poorly understood. It is unlikely that emergence delirium is related to the occurrence of the commonly seen excitatory EEG phenomena during induction. A direct change from an EEG pattern typical for anaesthesia to the awake-state EEG makes delirium likely; when it first changes to a normal sleep EEG the development of a delirium is unlikely. Anxiety at induction seems to be related with problematic behaviour on emergence, even with the old agent halothane (Aono *et al.* 1999). Similarly, soldiers with war experience are more prone to develop a delirium at awakening. Nevertheless, the author is convinced that this may present a different entity. Principally, delirium can occur in all age groups including adults (Card *et al.* 2015). It is very common, however, between the age of 6 months and 6 years. Very young babies commonly cry at emergence; but, when there is no pain, they can usually be consoled with a pacifier and sugar.

There are probably **no long-term consequences** of emergence delirium in children, e.g. negative behavioural changes; however, acutely, thrashing around could cause self-injury, loss of intravenous access and displacement of dressings. In addition, the parents are frightened because their usual strategies do not calm down the child, and additional work is created for the recovery room nurses. Therefore, every effort should be made to prevent emergence delirium.

There is a tremendous amount of literature focusing on the **prevention** of emergence delirium (Costi *et al.* 2014). Whereas premedication with midazolam and parental presence in the recovery room have no influence on the incidence of emergence delirium, alpha-2-agonists, opioids, ketamine and propofol are clearly effective. Improved emergence behaviour started the triumph of total intravenous anaesthesia (Lauder 2015). When inhalational anaesthesia is used, the emergence period has to be actively managed, e.g. by administering a dose of propofol at the end (Costi *et al.* 2015). A quietly sleeping preschool child is no guarantee that emergence delirium will not develop. Prophylactic medication can be omitted when the child is awake, responding to questions and aware of his or her surroundings. Whereas clear evidence exists on the prevention of emergence delirium, we have only expert opinions about **treatment** (Table 6.12). Opioids, ketamine and propofol are clearly effective; dexmedetomidine can be given with acceptable side effects as a bolus of 0.5 μg/kg. Even if it usually subsides spontaneously, emergence delirium has to be treated.

Summary and Recommendations

Emergence delirium is common in preschool children after a sevoflurane- or desflurane-based anaesthetic.

Table 6.12 The treatment of emergence delirium

Clinical situation	Compound	Comments
Pain or discomfort possible (e.g. ENT surgery)	Opioids	Nalbuphine in addition causes sedation
Severe agitation of unclear origin	Ketamine	Especially when opioids have already been tried
Pain unlikely (no surgery or a functioning regional block)	Propofol or thiopental	Propofol established, thiopental more reliable (?)
Airway patency critical	Dexmedetomidine	e.g. Cleft palate surgery when opioids have been given

Prophylactic medication is recommended in the susceptible age group. A quietly sleeping child at the end of surgery does not guarantee uneventful recovery.

In the case of emergence delirium, pain has to be excluded and/or treated first and therapeutic measures have to be taken; it is not good practice to let children cry.

References

Aono, J., Mamiya, K., & Manabe, M. (1999). Preoperative anxiety is associated with a high incidence of problematic behavior on emergence after halothane anesthesia in boys. *Acta Anaesthesiol Scand*, 43, 542–544.

Aono, J., Ueda, W., Mamiya, K., *et al.* (1997). Greater incidence of delirium during recovery from sevoflurane anesthesia in preschool boys. *Anesthesiology*, 87, 1298–1300.

Card, E., Pandharipande, P., Tomes, C., *et al.* (2015). Emergence from general anaesthesia and evolution of delirium signs in the post-anaesthesia care unit. *Br J Anaesth*, 115, 411–417.

Costi, D., Cyna, A.M., Ahmed, S., *et al.* (2014). Effects of sevoflurane versus other general anaesthesia on emergence agitation in children. *Cochrane Database Syst Rev*, (9), CD007084.

Costi, D., Ellwood, J., Wallace, A., *et al.* (2015). Transition to propofol after sevoflurane anesthesia to prevent emergence agitation: a randomized controlled trial. *Paediatr Anaesth*, 25, 517–523.

Cravero, J., Surgenor, S., & Whalen, K. (2000). Emergence agitation in paediatric patients after sevoflurane anaesthesia and no surgery: a comparison with halothane. *Paediatr Anaesth*, 10, 419–424.

Jöhr, M. (2002). Postanaesthesia excitation. *Paediatr Anaesth*, 12, 293–295.

Lauder, G.R. (2015). Total intravenous anesthesia will supercede inhalational anesthesia in pediatric anesthetic practice. *Paediatr Anaesth*, 25, 52–64.

Sikich, N. & Lerman, J. (2004). Development and psychometric evaluation of the pediatric anesthesia emergence delirium scale. *Anesthesiology*, 100, 1138–1145.

Somaini, M., Sahillioglu, E., Marzorati, C., *et al.* (2015). Emergence delirium, pain or both? A challenge for clinicians. *Paediatr Anaesth*, 25, 524–529.

7 Pre-existing Conditions

Malignant Hyperthermia

Case

Several decades ago, a 6-year-old girl, weighing 22 kg, was scheduled for adenotomy. With maternal presence, smooth anaesthesia induction was achieved with halothane and nitrous oxide. Venous access initially failed and, in the presence of a completely flaccid patient, the idea of endotracheal intubation without neuromuscular blockade came up. However, it was refused as being against the institutional policy. Venous access was ultimately successful and 30 mg (1.4 mg/kg) succinylcholine preceded by atropine 0.25 mg was injected. However, laryngoscopy was impossible, because of massive masseter rigidity. The anaesthetist called the supervising attending and mentioned malignant hyperthermia or myotonia as possible diagnoses. This was questioned by the attending, who proposed a second dose of succinylcholine. Finally, with some force, the trachea was successfully intubated.

The anaesthetist immediately requested a thermometer, which was not routinely available in theatre in those days, but the patient's legs felt as if they were made of wood when the nurse attempted to insert the rectal probe. Almost simultaneously, ventricular arrhythmias appeared at a heart rate of around 140 beats per minute. Malignant hyperthermia was now accepted by all team members as the presumptive diagnosis. The minute volume was increased and halothane was turned off. Fentanyl, droperidol and pancuronium were given. Dantrolene was requested and then given in a dose of 20 mg. An arterial blood sample taken at 10 minutes showed a metabolic acidosis and an already elevated creatine kinase (Table 7.1). Following two doses of 1.25 mg verapamil the arrhythmias disappeared and the heart rate gradually came down, the body temperature never rose, but fell from 36.8 °C to 36.0 °C. Two hours later adenotomy was performed. Then, once extubated, the girl voided a large quantity of reddish-brown urine. Because of shivering and peripheral cyanosis a second dose of 20 mg dantrolene was given.

Over the following hours, the body temperature rose to 38.5 °C, and after 24 hours creatine kinase peaked at 79 000 U/l. The girl suffered from transient muscle weakness and was discharged 2 weeks later with a letter stating the diagnosis of malignant hyperthermia.

Discussion

This case illustrates that **malignant hyperthermia (MH)** is an ever-present threat. Following a halothane induction, succinylcholine was a fulminant trigger for MH, initially presenting with masseter spasm, tachycardia and arrhythmias, followed by general muscle rigidity and rhabdomyolysis. With early treatment, cold infusions and exposure of the patient, an increase in body temperature could be prevented and was only seen later on the paediatric intensive care unit (PICU). Typically these patients, like the one described here,

Table 7.1 Blood chemistry during and following the anaesthetic

Time after onset of symptoms	10 min	60 min	150 min	6 h	24 h	48 h
pCO_2 (mmHg)	43	26	51			
pH	7.15	7.35	7.23			
Base excess	−14	−9.7	−6.7			
Na (mmol/l)	128		133			
K (mmol/l)	5.0		3.9			
Creatine kinase (U/l)	4876			21 000	79 000	48 900

have no noticeable abnormal phenotype, and creatine kinase values are within a normal range. Only four well-defined neuromuscular disorders are considered to be related with MH susceptibility (Klingler et al. 2009). These are central core disease, multi-minicore disease, nemaline rod myopathy and King–Denborough syndrome. The molecular basis of MH susceptibility is in most cases a mutation at the ryanodine-1 receptor (RYR1) gene located on chromosome 19, causing an uncontrolled release of intracellular calcium from the sarcoplasmic reticulum that induces a hypermetabolic state (Rosenberg et al. 2015). The elevated risk for rhabdomyolysis, e.g. in Duchenne muscular dystrophy (Veyckemans 2010), and the risk for a myotonic reaction in myotonia congenita (Parness et al. 2009) are different entities (Schieren et al. 2017).

The **diagnosis** is based on the **in vitro contracture** induced by halothane and caffeine in freshly biopsied muscle tissue. In addition, today, **molecular genetic** methods allow spotting mutations at the RYR1 gene. Therefore, when a mutation is found, a blood test allows a patient to be identified as at risk for developing a MH crisis. However, to exclude MH susceptibility, muscle biopsy is still needed, because it is likely that not all mutations are already known. Clinically many fewer cases are observed than one would expect, given the autosomal inheritance and the fact that genetically MH susceptibility may be as common as 1:3000. This phenomenon is poorly understood, as is the clear male predominance.

Modern **management of an MH crisis** is substantially different from the treatment used at the time of the case described here (Glahn et al. 2010). Today, the initial dose of dantrolene would have been 2.5 mg/kg, a dose that has been shown to stop an MH crisis; further dantrolene can be given up to a maximum of 10 mg/kg. Activated charcoal filters would probably have been applied at the inspiratory and the expiratory limbs of the circle. Exchanging the anaesthesia ventilator is no longer recommended. Laboratory investigation would have been made more often and at systematic time points, e.g. at the time of first suspicion, and then at 30 minutes, 4 hours, 12 hours and 24 hours, with a special focus on blood gas, lactate, potassium and myoglobin. It is likely that surgery would have been cancelled. Modern fluid therapy would have avoided the development of hyponatraemia with a sodium concentration of 128 mmol/l. Hyponatraemia was commonly seen in those days, when hypotonic solutions were routinely given during anaesthesia.

This charming patient accompanied the author through his whole professional life. Around a decade later, **malignant hyperthermia testing** became available in Switzerland. The family was contacted, and surprisingly the mother, who had experienced multiple uneventful anaesthetics in the 1970s, was found to be MH susceptible by muscle contracture testing. This is not an uncommon story; more than half of MH episodes are preceded by one or even several uneventful anaesthetics, and only 6.5% of the patients have a positive family history (Larach *et al.* 2010). Later, after **molecular genetic** workup, the responsible mutation was identified in this family, and when our patient gave birth to a son, the mutation was identified in the umbilical cord blood of the offspring (Girard *et al.* 2006).

Later in life, this patient had several uneventful anaesthetics. When so-called '**trigger-free anaesthesia**' is used, this means the avoidance of halogenated agents and succinylcholine, and a workplace that is adequately prepared (Cottron *et al.* 2014); the risk of an MH crisis is then abolished, and these patients can be treated and monitored as normal patients (Barnes *et al.* 2015).

Summary and Recommendations

Malignant hyperthermia (MH) is still with us, and every anaesthetist should be prepared to recognize the early signs of an MH episode.

Early treatment is crucial and dantrolene must be available. With timely treatment, an increase in body temperature may even be avoided altogether.

With 'trigger-free anaesthesia' these patients can be treated as normal patients. However, the workplace has to be adequately prepared.

References

Barnes, C., Stowell, K.M., Bulger, T., *et al.* (2015). Safe duration of postoperative monitoring for malignant hyperthermia patients administered non-triggering anaesthesia: an update. *Anaesth Intensive Care*, 43, 98–104.

Cottron, N., Larcher, C., Sommet, A., *et al.* (2014). The sevoflurane washout profile of seven recent anesthesia workstations for malignant hyperthermia-susceptible adults and infants: a bench test study. *Anesth Analg*, 119, 67–75.

Girard, T., Jöhr, M., Schaefer, C., *et al.* (2006). Perinatal diagnosis of malignant hyperthermia susceptibility. *Anesthesiology*, 104, 1353–1354.

Glahn, K.P., Ellis, F.R., Halsall, P.J., *et al.* (2010). Recognizing and managing a malignant hyperthermia crisis: guidelines from the European Malignant Hyperthermia Group. *Br J Anaesth*, 105, 417–420.

Klingler, W., Rueffert, H., Lehmann-Horn, F., *et al.* (2009). Core myopathies and risk of malignant hyperthermia. *Anesth Analg*, 109, 1167–1173.

Larach, M.G., Gronert, G.A., Allen, G.C., *et al.* (2010). Clinical presentation, treatment, and complications of malignant hyperthermia in North America from 1987 to 2006. *Anesth Analg*, 110, 498–507.

Parness, J., Bandschapp, O., & Girard, T. (2009). The myotonias and susceptibility to malignant hyperthermia. *Anesth Analg*, 109, 1054–1064.

Rosenberg, H., Pollock, N., Schiemann, A., *et al.* (2015). Malignant hyperthermia: a review. *Orphanet J Rare Dis*, 10, 93.

Schieren, M., Defosse, J., Böhmer, A., *et al.* (2017). Anaesthetic management of patients with myopathies. *Eur J Anaesthesiol*, 34, 641–649.

Veyckemans, F. (2010). Can inhalation agents be used in the presence of a child with myopathy? *Curr Opin Anaesthesiol*, 23, 348–355.

Case
7.2

Neuromuscular Disease

Case

Decades ago, a 14-year-old boy with Charcot–Marie–Tooth disease was scheduled for revision of the nail of the big toe because of chronic pain. After an inhalational induction, anaesthesia was maintained with sevoflurane in air and oxygen. For postoperative analgesia a toe block was performed with bupivacaine 0.75% using a 24G needle, and diclofenac was given. Primary surgery included partial removal of the nail, using the Kocher (or Emmert) procedure.

Despite an apparently functioning nerve block during surgery, postoperative pain was a major issue, even requiring opioid medication. Over the next few years repeated surgeries were performed. Severe postoperative pain and protracted healing occurred each time. In view of the underlying disease, the parents questioned the indication for the application of local anaesthetics, and their potential toxicity.

Discussion

This case of a child with a **neuromuscular disease**, an inherited peripheral neuropathy, provides an opportunity to emphasize several educational points.

First, the **classification** of neuromuscular diseases can be done according to the primary anatomical target: e.g. brain, spinal cord, nerve roots, peripheral nerve, neuromuscular junction or muscle cell. **Charcot–Marie–Tooth** (CMT) disease involves the peripheral nerves; it is most often an autosomal dominant inherited motor and sensory peripheral neuropathy, but a genetic heterogeneity of CMT exists. The onset of symptoms occurs usually around adolescence; however, as in this case, onset in childhood can also occur. In addition to muscle wasting and sensory loss, CMT can be associated with relevant extremity pain. Distal orthopaedic procedures, especially foot surgery to improve walking ability, are quite common in these patients. Over the later course of the disease, because of muscular weakness, a high risk of perioperative pulmonary complications is the predominant problem.

Second, **local anaesthetics** are not generally contraindicated in patients with neuromuscular disease (McSwain *et al.* 2014). Regional anaesthesia may even be a preferred technique, e.g. in patients at a high risk for pulmonary complications such as with myasthenia gravis (Kocum *et al.* 2007) or myotonic dystrophy (Tobias 1995). The author remembers a schoolboy with myotonic dystrophy who could be perfectly managed with a spinal block for orthopaedic surgery (Fig. 7.2). In patients with CMT disease, central neuraxial (Schmitt *et al.* 2004) as well as peripheral conduction blocks (Schmitt *et al.* 2014) have been used without any reports of neurologic deterioration. No information is available, however, about small peripheral nerves which are 'bathed' in a local anaesthetic solution, as was

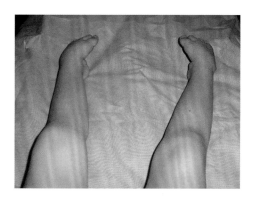

Figure 7.2 A child with myotonic dystrophy presenting for orthopaedic surgery.

the case in this patient with a toe block. Maybe these nerves are more vulnerable in the presence of pre-existing demyelinization and axon loss. In any case, a careful discussion with parents and patient about the risks and benefits of such a procedure is needed.

Third, in the context of neuromuscular diseases the use of **muscle relaxants** is of special interest. **Succinylcholine** can cause hyperkalaemia in patients with extensive paresis, e.g. paraplegia or Guillain–Barré disease; in children with Duchenne disease it triggers rhabdomyolysis (cf. Case 5.2). In patients with myotonic dystrophy or myotonia congenita a generalized myotonic reaction is feared, and succinylcholine is contraindicated too. Malignant hyperthermia (MH) is rarely a problem; only four well-defined entities are at an increased risk for MH (cf. Case 7.1). With **non-depolarizing relaxants** an altered sensibility and the risk of residual paralysis should be considered; e.g. in children with Duchenne disease (Muenster *et al.* 2006). Especially in children with pronounced muscle weakness, even minimal residual paralysis can be fatal; the use of rocuronium followed by sugammadex is nowadays established and even becoming the gold standard in such situations (Tobias 2017).

Fourth, in some diseases it is not only the neuromuscular system that is affected, but also other organs, such as the heart or the gastrointestinal tract (Veyckemans & Scholtes 2013). In particular, patients with myotonic dystrophy and Duchenne disease are at a high risk of cardiac complications.

Summary and Recommendations

This case of a child with Charcot–Marie–Tooth (CMT) disease illustrates that even if the literature does not provide any information about neurologic sequelae after regional anaesthesia, a careful risk–benefit analysis has to be made on an individual basis.

The use of rocuronium followed by sugammadex combines the benefits of a profound blockade during intubation and surgery with the absence of any residual paralysis after the intervention.

References

Kocum, A., Sener, M., Bozdogan, N., *et al.* (2007). Spinal anesthesia for inguinal hernia repair in 8-year-old child with myasthenia gravis. *Paediatr Anaesth*, 17, 1220–1221.

McSwain, J.R., Doty, J.W., & Wilson, S.H. (2014). Regional anesthesia in patients with pre-existing neurologic disease. *Curr Opin Anaesthesiol*, 27, 538–543.

Muenster, T., Schmidt, J., Wick, S., *et al.* (2006). Rocuronium 0.3 mg x kg-1 (ED95) induces a normal peak effect but an altered time course of neuromuscular block in patients with Duchenne's muscular dystrophy. *Paediatr Anaesth*, 16, 840–845.

Schmitt, H.J., Huberth, S., Huber, H., *et al.* (2014). Catheter-based distal sciatic nerve block in patients with Charcot–Marie–Tooth disease. *BMC Anesthesiol*, 14, 8.

Schmitt, H.J., Münster, T., & Schmidt, J. (2004). Central neural blockade in Charcot–

Marie–Tooth disease. *Can J Anaesth*, 51, 1049–1050.

Tobias, J.D. (1995). Anaesthetic management of the child with myotonic dystrophy: epidural anaesthesia as an alternative to general anaesthesia. *Paediatr Anaesth*, 5, 335–338.

Tobias, J.D. (2017). Current evidence for the use of sugammadex in children. *Paediatr Anaesth*, 27, 118–125.

Veyckemans, F. & Scholtes, J.L. (2013). Myotonic dystrophies type 1 and 2: anesthetic care. *Paediatr Anaesth*, 23, 794–803.

Case

Many decades ago, a 6-year-old girl with Down syndrome, weighing 28 kg, was scheduled for dental treatment. The history included repair of a ventricular septum defect at the age of 2 years and several attacks of 'asthma' which apparently responded to classic treatment. Anaesthesia was induced with etomidate, succinylcholine and halothane. Nasotracheal intubation with a size 6.0 uncuffed tube failed. Smaller tubes were tried, but finally only a size 3.0 uncuffed tube could be inserted orally, and no leak was present. After consultation with an ENT specialist the decision was made to postpone the intervention and to proceed to tracheotomy on the dental chair.

The girl was transferred to the paediatric intensive care unit (PICU). Tracheoscopy showed an almost circular subglottic stenosis which was seen as a sequela of cardiac surgery with prolonged postoperative ventilation. Consequently a laser resection of the stenosis was performed and a Montgomery T-tube was inserted to keep the lumen open. The patient, initially scheduled for outpatient dental treatment, stayed in hospital for over 3 months; during this stay the dental treatment was performed. The patient was discharged with the T-tube in situ. Many weeks later decannulation was successful and the further course was uneventful.

Discussion

This case of a girl with **Down syndrome** and unrecognized subglottic stenosis illustrates that symptoms of a disease are often not recognized in children who are 'special' and do not pass the normal steps of development as usual. It is very likely that the 'asthma' attacks represented the airway restriction caused by the stenosis, and that the reduced activity, or limited exercise tolerance, was related to the presence of Down syndrome and the previous cardiac surgery. Similar cases have been reported in the literature (Farrow & Guruswamy 2008). Syndromic children are always more likely to have an unrecognized pathology.

Down syndrome is associated with a variety of pathologies (Lewanda *et al.* 2016) putting these patients at an increased risk of **perioperative complications** (Borland *et al.* 2004), e.g. bradycardia, post-extubation stridor and airway obstruction. Also, postoperatively, there is a higher risk of respiratory depression (Jay *et al.* 2017); this is probably related to the difficulty in finding the correct dose and not to real pharmacokinetic or pharmacodynamic differences. The author remembers a fatality, many decades ago, in a child with Down syndrome who was on a morphine infusion 2 days after cleft palate repair.

Congenital heart disease is common in children with Down syndrome; but gastrointestinal malformations, e.g. duodenal atresia, and other conditions such as Hirschsprung disease and cleft palate are more common too. Malformations of the cardiovascular system are present in more than one-third of children with Down syndrome; the most common finding is an atrioventricular septal defect, as in our patient. A typical finding is **bradycardia** during a sevoflurane induction which is unrelated to hypoxaemia or overdose. The origin and significance of the phenomenon are still unclear, although it seems to be transient and is usually no longer present during maintenance. It was the author's practice just to observe bradycardia and not to treat it, because at the time of airway insertion it usually disappeared. Bradycardia was first mentioned in case reports (Roodman *et al.* 2003) and then systematically evaluated (Kraemer *et al.* 2010). Dexmedetomidine, which is known to cause bradycardia, can be given for sedation without an exaggerated risk (Miller *et al.* 2017). It is anyway an attractive choice in the view of the high incidence of airway obstruction and obstructive sleep apnoea in this population. **Pulmonary hypertension** is more common in children with Down syndrome and poses a major risk factor for general anaesthesia.

Children with Down syndrome typically have **airway problems**, not only obstructive sleep apnoea but also subglottic stenosis and other pathologies (Hamilton *et al.* 2016). They typically have smaller airway dimensions, and at the time when uncuffed tubes were exclusively used, it was recommended to start by using an endotracheal tube two sizes smaller than predicted by the age of the patient (Shott 2000). Today, for many routine interventions, all these considerations can be bypassed by using a laryngeal mask airway. Obstructive sleep apnoea is a very common feature; midface hypoplasia, pharyngeal muscle hypotonia, small airway dimensions combined with a relatively large tongue, obesity, increased secretions and common infections all contribute to the difficulties.

Craniocervical instability has a high incidence of up to over 60% in patients with Down syndrome; it involves the occiput–C1 level and more commonly the C1–C2 (atlantoaxial) level and is mostly seen in the context of generalized ligamentous laxity (Hata & Todd 2005). Forceful laryngoscopy and prolonged surgery with the head in the non-neutral position may put the patient at risk of a spinal cord injury. A preoperative radiographic screening in all patients with Down syndrome to exclude craniocervical instability is not realistic, and not requested by the majority of paediatric anaesthetists; every year thousands of such patients undergo anaesthesia without any problem. In symptomatic patients, however, further investigations and specialist advice should be requested. Chronic craniocervical instability can lead to a cervical myelopathy. The author remembers a 12-year-old girl whose ability to ambulate worsened over time despite corrective foot surgery, and who finally presented with a cervical myelopathy (Fig. 7.3).

Especially in the neonate with Down syndrome the **haematological peculiarities** have to be known. Neutrophilia is very common, and up to 10% have a transient myeloproliferative disorder. Polycythaemia and thrombocytopenia are additional features.

Children with Down syndrome present a challenge for the paediatric anaesthetist because of the associated pathologies and the sometimes reduced cooperation in association with reduced intellectual capacity. It has to be emphasized, however, that children with Down syndrome are the **sunshine in a paediatric hospital**, and almost all of them are loved by their caregivers because of their amiability.

Summary and Recommendations

Children with Down syndrome often have multiple associated pathologies; some of them may be unknown at the time of anaesthesia, as was the airway stenosis in this case.

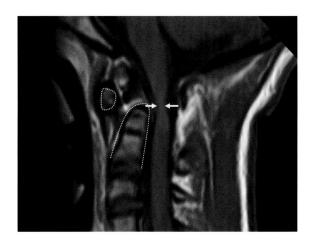

Figure 7.3 A MRI showing severe cervical myelopathy as a consequence of atlantoaxial instability in a 12-year-old girl.

Difficulties in airway management and the high likelihood of postoperative airway obstruction have to be anticipated.

The anaesthetist must be aware of the high incidence of congenital heart disease and the occurrence of transient bradycardia during sevoflurane induction.

References

Borland, L.M., Colligan, J., & Brandom, B.W. (2004). Frequency of anesthesia-related complications in children with Down syndrome under general anesthesia for noncardiac procedures. *Paediatr Anaesth*, 14, 733–738.

Farrow, C. & Guruswamy, V. (2008). Undiagnosed tracheal stenosis in a patient with Down's syndrome. *Paediatr Anaesth*, 18, 577.

Hamilton, J., Yaneza, M.M., Clement, W.A., et al. (2016). The prevalence of airway problems in children with Down's syndrome. *Int J Pediatr Otorhinolaryngol*, 81, 1–4.

Hata, T. & Todd, M.M. (2005). Cervical spine considerations when anesthetizing patients with Down syndrome. *Anesthesiology*, 102, 680–685.

Jay, M.A., Thomas, B.M., Nandi, R., et al. (2017). Higher risk of opioid-induced respiratory depression in children with neurodevelopmental disability: a retrospective cohort study of 12 904 patients. *Br J Anaesth*, 118, 239–246.

Kraemer, F.W., Stricker, P.A., Gurnaney, H.G., et al. (2010). Bradycardia during induction of anesthesia with sevoflurane in children with Down syndrome. *Anesth Analg*, 111, 1259–1263.

Lewanda, A.F., Matisoff, A., Revenis, M., et al. (2016). Preoperative evaluation and comprehensive risk assessment for children with Down syndrome. *Paediatr Anaesth*, 26, 356–362.

Miller, J., Ding, L., Spaeth, J., et al. (2017). Sedation methods for transthoracic echocardiography in children with trisomy 21: a retrospective study. *Paediatr Anaesth*, 27, 531–539.

Roodman, S., Bothwell, M., & Tobias, J.D. (2003). Bradycardia with sevoflurane induction in patients with trisomy 21. *Paediatr Anaesth*, 13, 538–540.

Shott, S.R. (2000). Down syndrome: analysis of airway size and a guide for appropriate intubation. *Laryngoscope*, 110, 585–592.

Oncologic Disease

Case

Many years ago, a 14-month-old girl, weighing 9 kg, was scheduled for the resection of a large abdominal neuroblastoma, bone marrow aspiration and portacath implantation. Anaesthesia was induced with 3 mg/kg ketamine, 10 µg/kg fentanyl and 0.6 mg/kg atracurium. For maintenance, isoflurane, an atracurium infusion and repeated doses of fentanyl up to a total dose of 30 µg/kg were given. In addition, before surgery, a caudal block with bupivacaine 0.25% and 50 µg/kg morphine had been performed. Two peripheral venous lines, a 4F double-lumen central venous catheter via the left subclavian vein and a femoral artery catheter, were in place.

After induction, the first non-invasively measured blood pressure was 150/70 mmHg. Despite isoflurane and several doses of fentanyl, blood pressure remained high and even peaked at 205/120 mmHg (Fig. 7.4). Only sodium nitroprusside and seven doses of 0.1 mg/kg labetalol brought some control. After tumour resection, hypotension immediately developed. The blood pressure could be maintained at 60/30 mmHg by the administration of 20 ml/kg of albumin, dopamine and noradrenaline. At the end of the anaesthetic, lasting 7 hours in all, the vasoactive support could be reduced and the further postoperative course was uneventful.

Discussion

This case gives a view of the 'early days' of paediatric oncology, when abdominal tumours, such as neuroblastoma or nephroblastoma, underwent primary resection which was only then followed by the oncologic treatment. The anaesthetist was adequately prepared for this type of surgery, often connected with major blood loss, perhaps with the exception that the femoral artery tracing was in danger of being lost during clamping of the abdominal aorta.

This case of **neuroblastoma** also illustrates that a careful preoperative workup is important; in such patients this should include checking blood pressure and the catecholamine values in blood and urine (Fujimura *et al.* 1992). In **phaeochromocytoma**, a rare disease in children (Hack 2000), hypertension is regularly seen and the accepted practice is preoperative medication with an adrenergic blocking agent, e.g. phenoxybenzamine, in order to avoid the dangerous intraoperative swings of blood pressure. Neuroblastoma is much more common in children; however, although the majority of these tumours secrete catecholamines, only a few of these patients (3–17%) present with intraoperative hypertension (Creagh-Barry & Sumner 1992, Haberkern *et al.* 1992). Nevertheless, the paediatric anaesthetist should be aware of the potential for severe intraoperative hypertension in neuroblastoma patients too (Haberkern *et al.* 1992, Kako *et al.* 2013, Seefelder *et al.*

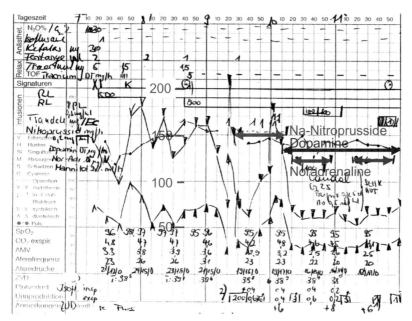

Figure 7.4 The chart of this 14-month-old child with a neuroblastoma presenting with massive hypertension.

2005). Some selective patients should perhaps be prepared in a similar manner to phaeo-chromocytoma. The same may be true for the extremely rare children with paraganglioma.

While taking care of the **oncologic child**, the anaesthetist should generally consider a number of points.

First, whether caused by the disease or by the anticancer chemotherapy, these patients are extremely susceptible to infections. **Perfect hygiene** and minimal tissue trauma (because of impaired healing) are of paramount importance.

Second, **anticancer medications** and irradiation may have long-term side effects, e.g. anthracycline-induced cardiotoxicity, which may be progressive and irreversible (Bansal *et al.* 2017), or vincristine-induced neuropathy.

Third, dexamethasone, which is commonly given for prevention of vomiting, may induce a life-threatening **tumour lysis syndrome**, even after a single dose (Sinha *et al.* 2009). In general, there is never a place in medicine for a 'routine medication' to every patient without challenging the indication.

Fourth, a bulky tumour in the anterior mediastinum can cause a **mediastinal mass syndrome** (Hack *et al.* 2008). With the loss of spontaneous ventilation, the decrease in functional residual capacity as well as venous congestion and increased pulmonary resistance caused by positive-pressure ventilation can provoke a cardiovascular collapse. The key feature is compression of the pulmonary outflow tract in addition to compression of the central air-conducting system. Pre-existing stridor and compression of the trachea cross-sectional area to less than 30% are predictors for complications. The best way is to avoid anaesthesia with controlled ventilation at all before a tumour-shrinking therapy has been initiated. In case of decompensation, lifting the sternum with a surgical forceps can be life-saving.

Fifth, children with tumours are **'frequent flyers'**, often presenting numerous times for imaging procedures or interventions. A procedure adapted to the child, providing high quality of care, ideally delivered each time by the same person, is of particular importance.

Summary and Recommendations

This case of neuroblastoma presenting with massive hypertension emphasizes the importance of being familiar with all aspects of the specific disease.

Typical features of the oncologic child should always be kept in mind: the side effects of anticancer medications, tumour lysis syndrome and mediastinal mass syndrome.

The oncologic child presenting repeatedly for interventions, and the parents, should perceive the anaesthetist as a good friend providing security and comfort in a difficult period of life.

References

Bansal, N., Amdani, S., Lipshultz, E.R., *et al.* (2017). Chemotherapy-induced cardiotoxicity in children. *Expert Opin Drug Metab Toxicol*, 13, 817–832.

Creagh-Barry, P. & Sumner, E. (1992). Neuroblastoma and anaesthesia. *Paediatr Anaesth*, 2, 147–152.

Fujimura, H., Kitamura, S., Kawahara, R., *et al.* (1992). Serum catecholamine concentrations and hemodynamics during operations on 23 children with neuroblastoma [in Japanese]. *Masui*, 41, 919–924.

Haberkern, C.M., Coles, P.G., Morray, J.P., *et al.* (1992). Intraoperative hypertension during surgical excision of neuroblastoma. Case report and review of 20 years' experience. *Anesth Analg*, 75, 854–858.

Hack, H.A. (2000). The perioperative management of children with phaeochromocytoma. *Paediatr Anaesth*, 10, 463–476.

Hack, H.A., Wright, N.B., & Wynn, R.F. (2008). The anaesthetic management of children with anterior mediastinal masses. *Anaesthesia*, 63, 837–846.

Kako, H., Taghon, T., Veneziano, G., *et al.* (2013). Severe intraoperative hypertension after induction of anesthesia in a child with a neuroblastoma. *J Anesth*, 27, 464–467.

Seefelder, C., Sparks, J.W., Chirnomas, D., *et al.* (2005). Perioperative management of a child with severe hypertension from a catecholamine secreting neuroblastoma. *Paediatr Anaesth*, 15, 606–610.

Sinha, R., Bose, S., & Subramaniam, R. (2009). Tumor lysis under anesthesia in a child. *Acta Anaesthesiol Scand*, 53, 131–133.

Case 7.5

The Diabetic Child

Case

Many years ago, a 6-year-old syndromic girl with craniosynostosis, weighing 16 kg, was scheduled for cranioplasty with the application of external distraction devices. After an inhalational induction and endotracheal intubation, anaesthesia was maintained with sevoflurane, repeated doses of fentanyl and a mivacurium infusion. Over the procedure, which lasted several hours, blood loss was replaced and repeated blood samples were taken, with the focus on haemoglobin and acid–base balance. The elevated glucose concentration, repeatedly measured as close to 20 mmol/l (360 mg/dl), was attributed to perioperative stress and the co-administration of dexamethasone and too much glucose. Similarly, on the paediatric intensive care unit (PICU), elevated glucose levels triggered a reduction of the glucose administration rate.

Later, on the ward, glucose remained at 10 mmol/l (180 mg/dl). But, because the focus was on the good surgical result, the patient was discharged home with a recommendation to the family physician that the glucose concentration should be checked at some point. A few weeks later the patient was admitted with a severe, life-threatening ketoacidotic derangement. Only now was the diagnosis of type 1 diabetes made.

Discussion

This case of missed diagnosis of childhood **diabetes**, despite repeated high glucose levels as an early warning sign, illustrates the importance of awareness of the disease. Diabetes is a relatively common disease in children with an incidence of 1:450 in the UK. In 97% it is type 1 diabetes (Ali *et al.* 2011), which is purely a hormonal deficiency syndrome. Type 2 diabetes occurs only occasionally, mostly in older children and in the context of syndromic entities or the erupting epidemic of childhood obesity. In children below 4 years of age, secondary enuresis is the first clinical sign in 89%, followed by the classic symptoms of polyuria, polydipsia and weight loss. The diagnosis is often missed initially, as in this case, and 30% of the children have at least one medical visit before the final diagnosis is made. Therefore, any isolated glucose measurement over 11 mmol/l (200 mg/dl) should initiate an investigation on the same day. This should include a careful history, measuring glucose and HbA_{1C} as well as planning a follow-up.

The management of diabetes involves more than just focusing on the abnormal glucose concentration. **Insulin is an anabolic hormone**; its functions include energy storage, transport functions and the protection of the 'stores', e.g. by the inhibition of lipolysis and gluconeogenesis. This latter function is preserved in type 2 diabetes, whereas in uncontrolled type 1 diabetes severe ketoacidosis is the usual fate. Insulin does much more than regulate the plasma glucose concentration. Especially in the perioperative period, where starvation is common, the increase in plasma glucose may be only moderate, but nevertheless protein catabolism, lipolysis and ketone production still occur. Therefore it is important to look beyond plasma glucose control; insulin and glucose administration are both needed.

The principles of modern **treatment** include providing a continuous basal level of insulin by the administration of long-acting insulin or the use of an insulin pump combined with smaller more frequent boluses of a very short-acting insulin. Diabetology is no hard science, and most recommendations are based on expert opinion (Rhodes *et al.* 2005, 2014). In the perioperative period the following points should be considered.

First, we should **optimize control** before surgery, focusing on absent ketonuria, normal serum electrolytes and HbA_{1C} close to the normal limits, ideally below 7.5%.

Second, we should **minimize starvation**, minimize 'cellular starvation' by the administration of glucose and insulin, reduce the stress response as much as possible and monitor the blood glucose concentration during anaesthesia at least every 60 minutes. Promoting early oral intake and avoiding postoperative vomiting should be among the anaesthetist's priorities.

Third, because of the risk of **unrecognized hypoglycaemia** in the anaesthetized patient, the blood glucose target should not be too low. During anaesthesia 5–10 mmol/l (90–180 mg/dl) and in the awake patient 4.5–8 mmol/l (80–160 mg/dl) are commonly recommended limits.

Fourth, for **major procedures** with an indefinite postoperative fasting period, morning insulin is withheld, glucose is monitored and an infusion of glucose and insulin is started (Table 7.5). As a rule of thumb, a child needs 2–3 mg/kg/min glucose, an adolescent 1–2 mg/kg/min. A more versatile approach is to infuse a balanced salt solution and glucose (e.g. 40%) in parallel. For **minor surgery**, patients on a basal-bolus regime or on an insulin pump receive the long-acting insulin as usual (perhaps reduced by 25%) or are kept on the basal rate. In addition, 2–3 mg/kg/min glucose is administered. However, according to the 2014 guidelines (Rhodes *et al.* 2014) fluids without glucose can be given too. With an appropriately titrated basal rate and careful monitoring, this approach may even be more physiological. Today, at least in Switzerland, the majority of recently diagnosed children

Table 7.5 A proposal for the administration of insulin and glucose (when fluids are given at a maintenance rate) in the context of major surgery leading to a prolonged period of postoperative fasting

0.5 U/kg regular insulin in 50 ml NaCl 0.9% 1 ml = 0.01 U/kg				
Glucose		Insulin		Fluid*
mmol/l	mg/dl	ml/h	U/kg/h	
15	> 270	10	0.1	Saline
8–15	146–269	5	0.05	Glucose 5%
4–8	80–145	5	0.05	Glucose 10%
< 4	< 80	2	0.02	Glucose 10%

* A more versatile approach is to infuse a balanced salt solution and a concentrated glucose solution (e.g. 40%) in parallel.

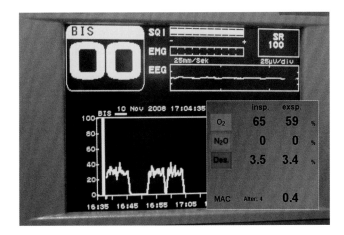

Figure 7.5 Patients with ketoacidosis may be very fragile. Burst-suppression EEG in a child during general anaesthesia for establishing vascular access despite only 0.4 MAC of desflurane.

with type 1 diabetes are treated with an insulin pump, some of them even combined with continuous glucose monitoring.

The cornerstone of treating **diabetic ketoacidosis** is fluids, insulin, potassium supplementation and later glucose administration (Wolfsdorf *et al.* 2014). Diabetic ketoacidosis can still kill, mainly by brain oedema, the pathophysiology of which is poorly understood. Anaesthetists must restrain their natural instincts and remember that, in this situation, fluids should not be given too fast or in excess. A balanced salt solution or normal saline are initially given at a rate of 10 ml/kg/h over the first 1–2 hours. A higher infusion rate of 20 ml/kg/h should only exceptionally be used for a short period in children presenting in circulatory shock. Then, for the next 24 hours, the rate of administration is reduced to the maintenance rate plus the estimated deficit (usually 5% of body weight). The amount of fluid administered over 24 hours should only exceptionally exceed twice the calculated maintenance rate. Surprisingly, normal saline is still widely used, leading to persisting acidosis, caused by hyperchloraemia (Taylor *et al.* 2006). Patients with ketoacidosis or other severe metabolic derangements may be very fragile; a reduced anaesthetic requirement is commonly seen (Fig. 7.5).

Summary and Recommendations

In the diabetic child the focus should be on more than just plasma glucose concentration; simultaneous administration of insulin and glucose is important.

Timely diagnosis of childhood diabetes is crucial; even a single measurement of glucose concentration over 11 mmol/l (200 mg/dl) should trigger an investigation on the same day.

Diabetic ketoacidosis requires a well-titrated treatment; correcting derangements too fast and too much can be lethal.

References

Ali, K., Harnden, A., & Edge, J.A. (2011). Type 1 diabetes in children. *BMJ*, 342, d294.

Rhodes, E.T., Ferrari, L.R., & Wolfsdorf, J.I. (2005). Perioperative management of pediatric surgical patients with diabetes mellitus. *Anesth Analg*, 101, 986–999.

Rhodes, E.T., Gong, C., Edge, J.A., *et al.* (2014). ISPAD Clinical Practice Consensus

Guidelines 2014. Management of children and adolescents with diabetes requiring surgery. *Pediatr Diabetes*, 15 (Suppl. 20), 224–231.

Taylor, D., Durward, A., Tibby, S.M., *et al.* (2006). The influence of hyperchloraemia on acid base interpretation in diabetic ketoacidosis. *Intensive Care Med*, 32, 295–301.

Wolfsdorf, J.I., Allgrove, J., Craig, M.E., *et al.* (2014). ISPAD Clinical Practice Consensus Guidelines 2014. Diabetic ketoacidosis and hyperglycemic hyperosmolar state. *Pediatr Diabetes*, 15 (Suppl. 20), 154–179.

Behavioural Disorders

Case

7.6

Case

Many years ago, a 10-year-old boy, weighing 30 kg, was scheduled for unilateral orchidopexy, which in those days was still performed as an inpatient procedure. The patient had been rescheduled a couple of times because of his fear as the day of surgery approached. Surgery was judged to be necessary, and psychological support was sought. Repeated sessions with the psychologist took place, and over time it came out that many months before he had experienced severe pain during the treatment of a fractured forearm, which had been done without anaesthetic support, with analgesia by nasal fentanyl alone. Before this experience he had never had a problem in medical surroundings.

On the day of surgery, the patient arrived on the ward accompanied by his parents and the psychologist, but he refused to swallow the planned heavy premedication consisting of 15 mg (0.5 mg/kg) midazolam and 150 mg (5 mg/kg) S-ketamine. So the nurse called the anaesthetist. In the discussion that followed, the normally developed and intelligent boy clearly recognized the need to have his testis moved into the scrotum, and that today was a good day for surgery because he was already here. His only fear was that when he took the first step and swallowed the premedication he would again be helpless and exposed to pain. The anaesthetist proposed the following procedure: no premedication to allow him to maintain complete control, walking together with mother and anaesthetist to the operating theatre, breathing the anaesthetic gases via a face mask, no needles or manipulations while awake, a guaranteed deep sleep because of brain monitoring (BIS) and good postoperative pain control.

The boy agreed, stood up, gave the mother a nod and accompanied the anaesthetist towards the door. At that point the psychologist intervened and said that this new plan would need further discussion. The anaesthetist lost his cool, the boy returned to his bed and surgery was cancelled.

Discussion

This patient developed an **anxiety disorder** based on an episode in the operating theatre where he felt abandoned and suffered severe pain. This reaction is understandable; the boy was determined that this should never happen to him again. This case also shows that honesty, pacing and leading are successful strategies, at least in a normally developed child. Keeping autonomy, e.g. walking to theatre and not being wheeled there on a trolley, is usually well accepted. Unfortunately, interruption of the flow and unprofessional behaviour obstructed the successful induction of anaesthesia.

This case also shows that, despite some progress in the prevention of pain in recent years, there is still **unnecessary suffering** in paediatric hospitals. Nasal opioids, e.g. fentanyl,

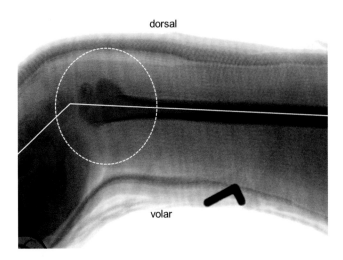

dorsal

volar

Figure 7.6 X-ray of the forearm, which had been brought into this position without anaesthesia. This was undoubtedly a painful procedure.

provide analgesia at rest in a child with a fractured forearm; but they will never be adequate for a fracture reduction. Some physicians erroneously believe that everything is OK during the placing of a cast and 'adjusting the position' of a fractured extremity, as long as the child does not cry or fight. However, some human beings in severe pain become immobile and lose their voice. Unfortunately the 'modern technologies', such as nasal opioids or nitrous oxide, are not always beneficial for children. Their effectiveness may be overestimated by the uninitiated practitioner, and so they create a **new category of victims** because physicians fail to request an anaesthetic.

In this case induction of anaesthesia was almost successful, until the psychologist stopped the flow. But the situation ran off the rails completely when the anaesthetist let his frustration show, always an inadequate behaviour. **Etiquette** (Kahn 2008), in this case maintaining poise in an annoying situation, is always valuable and part of professionalism (Becke & Jöhr 2017). One has to realize that, for the paediatric anaesthetist, guiding an uncooperative child towards a successful induction is a common experience, whereas for the psychologist the mere idea of entering the induction room herself may be distressing – as she has never experienced the mostly enjoyable atmosphere of a paediatric anaesthesia induction, which can even involve laughter and play. This specific episode initiated closer cooperation between the anaesthetic and psychological teams, and visits to the operating theatre were planned.

The **uncooperative child** is a big issue in paediatric anaesthesia. Major causes for being uncooperative are anxiety, mental overload and pain; in addition, a few children are simply ill-behaved or – rarely – have a mental illness. Early recognition is essential, because it is all about prevention. It is always good to win the parents' support; children benefit when they feel that their parents support the anaesthetist and have trust in what is going to happen. Anxiety and uncertainty are transferable from parents to children. Although parental presence has not been shown to reduce the child's anxiety (Wright et al. 2010), avoiding separation is beneficial and in the author's opinion clearly the way to go. A sedative premedication is helpful, and it does improve behaviour at induction (Cox et al. 2006). An induction with physical **restraint** should be the exception; however, it is unrealistic to require the abandonment of all forms of fixation and restraint; e.g. establishing venous access will need some form of immobilization in most if not all preschool children. There is a lively debate about this topic in the anaesthetic as well as in the paediatric literature (Homer & Bass 2010). The conclusion will probably be that the decision about what is considered tolerable will always depend on the indication and the applied force, e.g. using restraint in a normally developed teenager is probably unacceptable, whereas infants may routinely experience restraint during induction of anaesthesia. Finally, postponing anaesthesia can be an option, especially for older children with non-urgent surgery. Especially for uncooperative adolescents with reduced mental capacity, the anaesthetist may need an inventive mind; the author remembers children induced on the floor outside the operating theatre and even on the street in front of the paediatric hospital. However, this was always done with the full support of the parents, and the necessary precautions were taken.

In children with **attention deficit hyperactivity disorder** (ADHD) the risk for uncooperative behaviour at induction and for prolonged postoperative maladaptive behaviour is increased (Tait *et al.* 2010). It takes longer for these children to return to normal daily activity (Rosander *et al.* 2015). The administration of a heavy premedication, e.g. midazolam and ketamine, can be helpful; however, for some, especially for older and intellectually normal children, omitting premedication may be the better option in order not to destroy the last bit of self-control. Many of these children are under medication with stimulating drugs, e.g. methylphenidate. These drugs are highly effective and can be given preoperatively without any increased risk of adverse cardiovascular events (Cartabuke *et al.* 2017).

Autism spectrum disorder (ASD) is common, with a prevalence of 1%, and presents a major challenge to the paediatric anaesthetist (Taghizadeh *et al.* 2015). Deficits in social interaction and ritualistic repetitive behaviour are typical of children with ASD, and intellectual disability occurs in more than half of these patients. They may have difficulties in managing sensory inputs. As always, parents know best how their child will react in a certain situation. An individualized anaesthetic plan is required, and it should only be changed at short notice when unavoidable (Swartz *et al.* 2017). Heavy premedication is often required, and it is wise to make such a child the first patient on the surgical list.

Summary and Recommendations

The unwilling and uncooperative child requires an experienced anaesthetist who is able to adapt the proceedings to the special needs of the individual child.

Heavy premedication, postponing surgery and, very rarely, induction with physical restraint have to be discussed.

Professionalism requires etiquette, which includes maintaining poise in annoying situations.

References

Becke, K. & Jöhr, M. (2017). Etiquette, competence, and professionalism: the profile of the 'ideal pediatric anesthesiologist'. *Paediatr Anaesth*, 27, 116–117.

Cartabuke, R.S., Tobias, J.D., Rice, J., *et al.* (2017). Hemodynamic profile and behavioral characteristics during induction of anesthesia in pediatric patients with attention deficit hyperactivity disorder. *Paediatr Anaesth*, 27, 417–424.

Cox, R.G., Nemish, U., Ewen, A., *et al.* (2006). Evidence-based clinical update: does premedication with oral midazolam lead to improved behavioural outcomes in children? *Can J Anaesth*, 53, 1213–1219.

Homer, J.R. & Bass, S. (2010). Physically restraining children for induction of general anesthesia: survey of consultant pediatric anesthetists. *Paediatr Anaesth*, 20, 638–646.

Kahn, M.W. (2008). Etiquette-based medicine. *N Engl J Med*, 358, 1988–1989.

Rosander, S., Nause-Osthoff, R., Voepel-Lewis, T., *et al.* (2015). A comparison of the postoperative pain experience in children with and without attention-deficit hyperactivity disorder (ADHD). *Paediatr Anaesth*, 25, 1020–1025.

Swartz, J.S., Amos, K.E., Brindas, M., *et al.* (2017). Benefits of an individualized perioperative plan for children with autism spectrum disorder. *Paediatr Anaesth*, 27, 856–862.

Taghizadeh, N., Davidson, A., Williams, K., *et al.* (2015). Autism spectrum disorder (ASD) and its perioperative management. *Paediatr Anaesth*, 25, 1076–1084.

Tait, A.R., Voepel-Lewis, T., Burke, C., *et al.* (2010). Anesthesia induction, emergence, and postoperative behaviors in children with attention-deficit/hyperactivity disorders. *Paediatr Anaesth*, 20, 323–329.

Wright, K.D., Stewart, S.H., & Finley, G.A. (2010). When are parents helpful? A randomized clinical trial of the efficacy of parental presence for pediatric anesthesia. *Can J Anaesth*, 57, 751–758.

Anaphylaxis

Case

A 6-year-old boy, weighing 14 kg, was put on the emergency list because of an ileus with dilated bowel loops. According to the surgeon, only a short procedure was anticipated. The child's history included oesophageal and anal atresia necessitating several surgical interventions. On direct questioning the mother denied allergy or asthma.

Anaesthesia was induced uneventfully with propofol 4 mg/kg, alfentanil twice 15 μg/kg, rocuronium 0.7 mg/kg, and the child was intubated with a size 6.0 uncuffed endotracheal tube. Anaesthesia was maintained uneventfully with sevoflurane 2 V% in air and oxygen. The anaesthetist was looking at the multiple abdominal scars, and inserted an internal jugular catheter, while surgery had already started.

Suddenly the airway pressure alarmed and manual ventilation proved to be almost impossible, as if the Y-piece had been occluded with a thumb. There was no sign of dysfunction of the anaesthesia ventilator, a suction catheter passed the tube without difficulty, auscultation showed minimal to absent breath sounds on both sides, the radial pulse was very weak, and aspiration of the central venous catheter showed a normal return of blood without resistance. All mechanical reasons excluded, anaphylaxis with severe bronchospasm remained the most probable diagnosis. Adrenaline 100 μg, 30 μg and 100 μg (higher doses than currently recommended) were given intravenously, leading to almost immediate relief and allowing ventilation without resistance. In addition H_1 and H_2 blockers and an additional bolus of Ringer's lactate were given.

After uneventful surgery the child was extubated and transferred to the intensive care unit. Questioned again, the mother still denied allergy, but she mentioned that the child didn't like bananas, because they caused coughing. In addition the boy came home from school with a swollen face after contact with a rubber. There was no doubt about the diagnosis of latex allergy.

Discussion

This is a case of fulminant **latex allergy**, which became apparent as soon as the surgeon explored the abdomen with his gloves. The child had a typical history of multiple surgeries and subtle clues in the history: coughing while eating bananas, because tropical fruits can cross-react with latex, and the facial swelling after contact with a rubber at school. Interestingly, allergy was denied at direct questioning.

With the beginning of the HIV epidemic in the 1980s the whole population was exposed intensively to low-quality latex products, especially latex gloves. This triggered an epidemic of latex allergy (Gerber *et al.* 1989), which became the most common cause for an anaphylactic

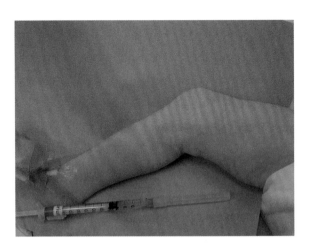

Figure 7.7 Cutaneous reaction following the injection of 0.2 mg/kg mivacurium, caused by direct histamine release.

reaction in children during anaesthesia (Murat 1993). Initially latex allergy was thought to be associated with spina bifida, but this is not the case; it is just exposure to repeated surgery (Porri *et al.* 1997). Sensitization also became a problem among medical personnel (Konrad *et al.* 1997). As a consequence, the medical community tried to reduce the use of latex-containing products, and especially the quality of the latex products was improved: they now release much less latex protein, and, without powder, the contact surface and the spread of latex particles is further reduced. Latex allergy is nowadays becoming rare (Blaabjerg *et al.* 2015). Therefore, for children with spina bifida, the classic latex-free treatment beginning at birth is no longer supported by all experts. Today, compounds other than latex are more likely to trigger anaphylaxis, e.g. antibiotics, colloids, muscle relaxants or chlorhexidine (Meng *et al.* 2017). The direct release of histamine caused by a drug, e.g. mivacurium or atracurium, is a different entity, not antibody-related and usually a benign phenomenon (Fig. 7.7). It can be diminished by reducing the dose and injecting slowly.

The **diagnosis** of latex allergy relies on the history of the child. If it remains unclear whether certain symptoms of instability are caused by an anaphylactic reaction, tryptase should be measured; it peaks at a time between 30 minutes and 3 hours. Serum can be frozen for later examination; post-mortem blood cannot be used. After an interval of 6 weeks the serum antibodies can be measured and skin tests can be performed. If it is done too early a negative test may not be diagnostic. Equally, a very late workup, e.g. after 2 or more years, is not recommended, because it may no longer be diagnostic. Years or even decades later, only a re-exposure test can give a definitive answer.

The key to successful **treatment** is the early administration of adrenaline (Dhami *et al.* 2014). Anaesthetists tend to administer drugs intravenously; however, in this situation intramuscular administration of adrenaline 10 μg/kg is preferable, as it provides much more reliable relief from the symptoms. After the intravenous administration of adrenaline 1 μg/kg, symptoms tend to reappear a few minutes later, as in this case. Of course, theoretically, a small bolus of adrenaline followed by a continuous infusion would be the optimal choice. But this is often not practical in these busy situations. Intramuscular adrenaline has been shown to be highly effective after cardiac arrest in an animal experiment (Mauch *et al.* 2013). In addition, corticosteroids and, probably less important, H_1 and H_2 blockers are given.

Summary and Recommendations

This case illustrates intraoperative anaphylaxis triggered by the latex of the surgical gloves. The most impressive clinical symptom was bronchospasm, which was rapidly relieved by the administration of adrenaline.

Adrenaline is the cornerstone of treatment; intramuscular administration of drugs is not very familiar to anaesthetists, but in the case of anaphylaxis intramuscular injection of adrenaline is the preferred treatment.

This case also shows that a firm statement by the parents that a child is not allergic does not preclude this diagnosis.

References

Blaabjerg, M.S., Andersen, K.E., Bindslev-Jensen, C., *et al.* (2015). Decrease in the rate of sensitization and clinical allergy to natural rubber latex. *Contact Dermatitis*, 73, 21–28.

Dhami, S., Panesar, S.S., Roberts, G., *et al.* (2014). Management of anaphylaxis: a systematic review. *Allergy*, 69, 168–175.

Gerber, A.C., Jörg, W., Zbinden, S., *et al.* (1989). Severe intraoperative anaphylaxis to surgical gloves: latex allergy, an unfamiliar condition. *Anesthesiology*, 71, 800–802.

Konrad, C., Fieber, T., Gerber, H., *et al.* (1997). The prevalence of latex sensitivity among anesthesiology staff. *Anesth Analg*, 84, 629–633.

Mauch, J., Ringer, S.K., Spielmann, N., *et al.* (2013). Intravenous versus intramuscular epinephrine administration during cardiopulmonary resuscitation: a pilot study in piglets. *Paediatr Anaesth*, 23, 906–912.

Meng, J., Rotiroti, G., Burdett, E., *et al.* (2017). Anaphylaxis during general anaesthesia: experience from a drug allergy centre in the UK. *Acta Anaesthesiol Scand*, 61, 281–289.

Murat, I. (1993). Anaphylactic reactions during paediatric anaesthesia: results of a survey of the French Society of Paediatric Anaesthetists (ADARPEF) 1991–1992. *Paediatr Anaesth*, 3, 339–343.

Porri, F., Pradal, M., Lemiere, C., *et al.* (1997). Association between latex sensitization and repeated latex exposure in children. *Anesthesiology*, 86, 599–602.

Case 7.8 Sepsis

Case

Several decades ago, a 3-month-old boy, weighing 3.8 kg, was brought by his parents to the emergency room of a district hospital because of high body temperature and reduced general condition. The previous day, the child had been seen by the local paediatrician for a routine check-up, and he had been vaccinated against diphtheria, tetanus and pertussis.

The physician on call was in his sixth year of postgraduate training including paediatrics and anaesthesia. He found a pale and hypotonic child with a body temperature of 40.5 °C. The child was tachypnoeic but no rales could be heard over the lungs and palpation of the abdomen did not seem to be painful. Inspection of the ears and the pharynx resulted in normal findings. The physician called the private paediatrician; he confirmed that the baby had been perfectly healthy the day before, and a vaccination reaction was the most likely diagnosis. Despite it being the weekend, he offered to see the family in his office if the situation did not improve.

Against fever, acetylsalicylic acid was given rectally and the child was discharged home. Several hours later the parents came rushing into the hospital carrying their dead child in their arms. Resuscitation was unsuccessful. Post-mortem examination was performed after a delay of more than 2 days; it did not reveal any specific disease. The final diagnosis was a lethal vaccination reaction. Many weeks later, the final medical report by the pathologist mentioned that there was also moderate growth of *Escherichia coli* in the cardiac blood.

Discussion

This case, which was not directly related to an anaesthetic, has heavily influenced the professional careers of the staff involved, and the way they practice medicine. It raises several educational points.

First, a **diagnosis** is never 100% certain; a vaccination reaction was only the most likely cause, and today a full blood count, blood gas, C-reactive protein, perhaps procalcitonin and urine sample would be required in a child with unexplained high fever. But in those days these examinations were not yet part of routine medical practice, or not available in the institution on an emergency basis. The author's personal conclusion is that if there is residual doubt about a diagnosis or even just a bad 'gut feeling' it is always worthwhile considering keeping a patient under closer supervision or organizing transfer to a specialized institution. This is particularly true for very young patients.

Second, **vaccination reactions** can occur, and it is relevant for the anaesthetist to know about a recent vaccination of the child. The current debate about vaccination and

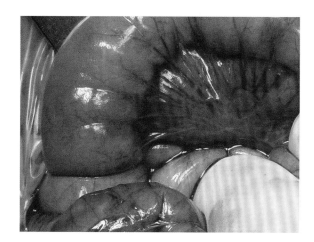

Figure 7.8 Intravascular gas bubbles in a septic preterm baby with an unfavourable outcome. Sepsis is a rapidly progressing disease and has to be treated without delay.

anaesthesia focuses on two points: the immunomodulatory influence of anaesthesia attenuating the immune response, and the vaccination reaction causing diagnostic uncertainty in the perioperative period. The current evidence does not provide any contraindication to immunization of children scheduled for elective surgery; however, respecting a minimum delay between vaccination and elective anaesthesia, e.g. 2 days for inactivated vaccines and 14–21 days for live attenuated viral vaccines, may avoid confounding of vaccine-caused events with postoperative complications (Siebert *et al.* 2007). The author has never postponed anaesthesia because of a recent vaccination, and has even accepted the wish of parents to vaccinate a child during anaesthesia – but only following a thorough discussion about the current controversy (Short *et al.* 2006).

Third, in a sick child, **sepsis** should always be included in the list of differential diagnoses. In a hospital setting, bacteraemia has been reported to be as common as 1:250 in febrile children under 5 years of age, but for the physician it is often difficult to recognize it without additional workup (Craig *et al.* 2010). In the described case, moderate growth of *Escherichia coli* in blood taken from an already autolytic cadaver, because the post-mortem examination was done after a delay of several days, was by no means proof of sepsis, and was judged at the time to be an insignificant finding. Nevertheless it still pops up in the minds of the staff involved when they recall the situation. Sepsis is a life-threatening disease (Fig. 7.8). Early recognition and adequate treatment are essential (Davis *et al.* 2017, Martin & Weiss 2015). A 'diagnostic bundle' and a 'treatment bundle' should be established on an institutional basis, so that no delay or uncertainty occurs. The antimicrobial treatment should be initiated without delay (Weiss *et al.* 2014): every hour counts. These general principles must be familiar to the paediatric anaesthetist. Cardiocirculatory stabilization is of course central to the role of the anaesthetist, but preoperatively and in emergency medicine he or she must also insist that timely antimicrobial therapy is initiated.

Summary and Recommendations

In a sick child, sepsis should always be included in the list of differential diagnoses. It is a life-threatening disease, and early recognition and treatment are essential.

In a recently vaccinated child, a vaccination reaction may cause fever and neurological symptoms. This has to be known by the anaesthetist, but there is no compelling evidence of a beneficial effect of postponing elective surgery.

If there is residual doubt about a smooth postoperative course or just a bad 'gut feeling', it is always worthwhile considering keeping the patient under closer supervision. Post-operatively, just go and have a look at the patient once more.

References

Craig, J.C., Williams, G.J., Jones, M., *et al.* (2010). The accuracy of clinical symptoms and signs for the diagnosis of serious bacterial infection in young febrile children: prospective cohort study of 15 781 febrile illnesses. *BMJ*, 340, c1594.

Davis, A.L., Carcillo, J.A., Aneja, R.K., *et al.* (2017). American College of Critical Care Medicine clinical practice parameters for hemodynamic support of pediatric and neonatal septic shock. *Crit Care Med*, 45, 1061–1093.

Martin, K. & Weiss, S.L. (2015). Initial resuscitation and management of pediatric septic shock. *Minerva Pediatr*, 67, 141–158.

Short, J.A., van der Walt, J.H., & Zoanetti, D.C. (2006). Immunization and anesthesia: an international survey. *Paediatr Anaesth*, 16, 514–522.

Siebert, J.N., Posfay-Barbe, K.M., Habre, W., *et al.* (2007). Influence of anesthesia on immune responses and its effect on vaccination in children: review of evidence. *Paediatr Anaesth*, 17, 410–420.

Weiss, S.L., Fitzgerald, J.C., Balamuth, F., *et al.* (2014). Delayed antimicrobial therapy increases mortality and organ dysfunction duration in pediatric sepsis. *Crit Care Med*, 42, 2409–2417.

Pregnancy

Case

Decades ago, a 16-year-old girl, weighing 60 kg, was scheduled for surgical revision because of an aching heel. One month earlier, she had gone to the general practitioner and asked for advice because of her foot. Three weeks ago, she entered the hospital as an inpatient, underwent physical examination, but was sent home following a decision taken at the office desk, because of an elevated sedimentation rate. But the general practitioner appealed for surgery to proceed, because the girl seemed to be suffering. So she was admitted to hospital again, underwent a 'thorough' physical examination, and was seen by an anaesthesiology trainee. She finally arrived in the operating theatre on the next day.

Following midazolam sedation, an experienced trainee inserted a lumbar epidural catheter and 20 ml of carbonated lidocaine 2% with adrenaline resulted, surprisingly, in a sensory level at T2. An anaesthetic nurse observed the patient in the induction room for some time, but finally called the senior supervising anaesthetist, because the theatre nurse claimed that the protruding abdomen prevented the patient from being positioned prone. The anaesthetist, who had been trained for more than a year in obstetrics, performed an external examination and diagnosed an advanced pregnancy with the fetus in breech position. A gynaecologist was urgently called to the OR for advice. Because of the young age and the innocent aspect of the schoolgirl he first assumed a large ovarian cyst and some ascites, but then the ultrasound examination confirmed the pregnancy. Because there was, still in the orthopaedic OR, some vaginal discharge followed by irregular contractions, the girl was transferred to the delivery suite, where a healthy term baby was delivered by urgent caesarean section on the same day.

Discussion

This case of **unrecognized pregnancy** in a teenage girl illustrates several educational points.

First, the **potential existence of pregnancy** has always to be considered in a girl beyond the age of menarche. The menstrual history and the age at menarche are often asked by the careful practitioner. But, understandably enough, most adults are reluctant to explore the sexual life of teenagers at a preoperative visit (Donaldson *et al.* 2012). Nevertheless, in selective cases, perhaps it should be done. Whereas in Switzerland and other countries it is considered the responsibility of patients and parents to disclose a potential pregnancy, in other places routine pregnancy testing is performed in every girl beyond a certain age, which may be as low as 11 years. However, in many populations, this would be considered almost an offence, and it seems to be sufficient just to offer testing only in cases of real uncertainty (Malviya *et al.* 1996). Anaesthesia and minor surgery during an unknown pregnancy would pose only a minimal risk to the fetus and the mother, but with other treatments, e.g. radiology or certain medications, this is certainly not the case.

Second, **medical charts may not necessarily tell the truth**. Even very obvious clinical signs may not be perceived by the patient or noticed by the physician. This girl, pregnant near term, was seen by four different physicians (the general practitioner, twice by a physician on the ward, and by the anaesthetist) and none of them saw anything unusual, because they did not expect it and were focusing only on the patient's heel. This patient even twice underwent a 'ritual' physical examination which included, according to the notes, palpation of the liver and the spleen. It is of paramount importance that anaesthetists approach every child with a completely open mind, expecting all kinds of surprises.

Third, this girl went to the general practitioner mainly to seek help, showing him her aching heel, but obviously this was not her main concern. Therefore, every conversation with patients and parents should include at least **one open question**, e.g. 'otherwise, how is life?' or 'is there anything else to discuss?' – thus giving them the chance to lead the conversation towards the real burning problems in their life. Getting into conversation with this patient was not at all difficult; she freely recounted her problems at school, the unwanted increase in body weight and also, on direct questioning, that she had had unprotected sexual intercourse. But, regrettably, no medical person wanted to hear this until she was lying on the operating table with an epidural extending to T2.

Fourth, during pregnancy the extension of an **epidural block** is increased by about one-third. In a non-pregnant 16-year-old girl a block extension only up to T10 would have been expected after the injection of 20 ml of 2% lidocaine. In a pregnant woman this volume is usually sufficient for a caesarean section. Another important factor is the age of the patient; the highest dose requirement is at the age of 18 years (Bromage 1969).

Although a proportion of teenage girls are taking **oral contraceptives**, paediatric anaesthetists are often not used to discussing this topic with their patients. The introduction of sugammadex into clinical practice (Tobias 2017), however, has made it more of a burning issue. Sugammadex not only encapsulates steroid muscle relaxants, but, to some extent, steroid hormones too, which reduces the reliability of hormonal contraceptives. An additional non-hormonal method of contraception should be recommended for this menstrual cycle, as is done when one dose of the contraceptive pill has been missed (Dalton & Van Hasselt 2016). This has to be made clear to the patients.

Summary and Recommendations

This case of unrecognized term pregnancy reminds us that every girl beyond menarche could potentially be pregnant.

Paediatric anaesthetists should be aware of girls taking hormonal contraceptives, at least when sugammadex is included in the anaesthetic management.

Anaesthetists should approach every child with a completely open mind, expecting all kinds of surprises, and every conversation should include an open question.

References

Bromage, P.R. (1969). Ageing and epidural dose requirements: segmental spread and predictability of epidural analgesia in youth and extreme age. *Br J Anaesth*, 41, 1016–1022.

Dalton, J. & Van Hasselt, G. (2016). Sugammadex: time of onset: nine months. *Anaesthesia*, 71, 115–116.

Donaldson, J.F., Napier, S.J., Ward-Jones, M., *et al.* (2012). Checking pregnancy status in adolescent girls before procedures under general anaesthesia. *Arch Dis Child*, 97, 895–899.

Malviya, S., D'Errico, C., Reynolds, P., *et al.* (1996). Should pregnancy testing be routine in adolescent patients prior to surgery? *Anesth Analg*, 83, 854–858.

Tobias, J.D. (2017). Current evidence for the use of sugammadex in children. *Paediatr Anaesth*, 27, 118–125.

8 Miscellaneous

Damage Caused by Pressure

Case

Many years ago, a 1 3/12-year-old boy, weighing 7 kg, with a history of preterm birth at 30 weeks of gestation and a birth weight of 600 g, was scheduled for proximal hypospadias repair. After an inhalational induction followed by the administration of 1.5 mg mivacurium he was nasotracheally intubated with a size 4.5 uncuffed tube. Anaesthesia was maintained with desflurane and a continuous infusion of mivacurium. A penile block with two paramedian injections of 0.7 ml bupivacaine 0.75% and a caudal block with 5 ml ropivacaine 0.2% and 2 µg/kg clonidine, preceded by an adrenaline-containing test dose, were performed. A 24G venous cannula was inserted into the left external jugular vein for repeated blood sampling and a BIS monitor was applied.

The anaesthetic course was uneventful over 6 hours with haemodynamic stability and constant respiratory parameters, except for a rise in body temperature which culminated 2 hours after induction at 39 °C. The temperature started to rise when the patient was fully covered by the surgical drapes with only the small surgical field exposed and was still actively warmed by a convective warming system. Because of the stable minute ventilation, malignant hyperthermia was considered to be unlikely. The active warming was stopped and the body temperature gradually came down. In addition, hourly blood gas measurements did not show acidosis or elevated lactate levels. At the end of the case a second caudal was performed, and the child was extubated and transferred to the paediatric intensive care unit (PICU) for further observation.

Just to be on the safe side, creatine kinase (CK) was measured; it was 479 U/l (normal value < 195 U/l) and culminated after 24 hours at 928 U/l. The clinical examination showed a peacefully sleeping child with a normal respiratory rate and a warm periphery. However, the left calf was impressively indurated. Analysis identified continuous pressure applied by the surgical assistant as the most probable causative factor for this localized muscle damage (Fig. 8.1a).

Discussion

This case of **rhabdomyolysis caused by pressure** illustrates the importance of paying meticulous attention to every detail. Staff not regularly involved in the care of small children, in this case a young surgical trainee, often forget that under the drapes lies a small human body and are often unaware how frail a small child can be. Anaesthetists usually immediately ask for a change when surgical colleagues are compressing the thorax and interfering with ventilation. But the anaesthetist should have a synoptic view of the perioperative process, and should give immediate advice if

(a)

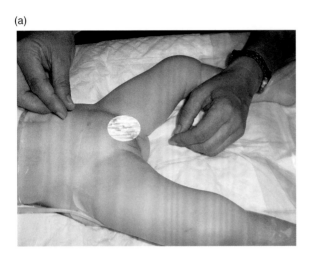

Figure 8.1a Re-staged situation during hypospadias surgery: pressure from the surgical assistant's forearm caused localized rhabdomyolysis.

something does not seem to be in the best interest of the patient, even if not directly related to anaesthesia.

Surgery leads to some **increase in creatine kinase**. In children after minor surgery values of 15–195 U/l have been found, after major surgery 58–770 U/l (Yousef *et al.* 2006). In adults even higher values, in some case over 1000 U/l, can occur (Laurence 2000). The increase depends on the extent and duration of surgery (Mouzopoulos *et al.* 2007). CK usually peaks on the first postoperative day. In the reported case the increase in CK was far beyond the expected range caused by penile surgery in a child, where no muscle is cut or squeezed at all. Blood pressure monitoring over a prolonged time can also induce muscle (Srinivasan & Kuppuswamy 2012) or nerve damage (Swei *et al.* 2009). It is probably unwise to select a very short cycle time over a prolonged period when it is not absolutely needed. In this case the blood pressure cuff was applied on the upper extremity.

The **surgical positioning** can enhance rhabdomyolysis by a combination of direct pressure on the muscle and a position-dependent low perfusion pressure. This occurs typically with an extreme head-down lithotomy position and has been reported in children too (Bocca *et al.* 2002). The length of surgery is a relevant factor (Poli *et al.* 2007). The author remembers a girl who developed severe tenderness of both lower legs followed by muscle weakness, walking difficulties and long-term sequelae after prolonged transanal colorectal surgery in the lithotomy position.

Much more common in daily practice are pressure sores or even localized **skin necrosis** caused by insufficient padding of a peripheral venous access device (Fig. 8.1b) or a splint for immobilization of the extremity. Because of the high rate of pressure sores in the region of the calcaneus, even when rigorous standards are followed, the author gave up using a splint for the immobilization of a venous access on the foot.

Pressure injuries from pulse oximeter sensors that are too tightly attached regularly occur (Ceran *et al.* 2012), especially when the sensor is secured before induction in an awake struggling child. It is recommended to re-attach the sensor after induction under well-controlled conditions when the child is no longer trying actively to remove it.

(b)

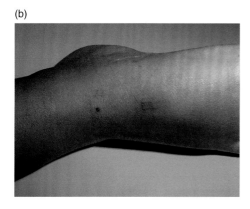

Figure 8.1b Skin necrosis caused by an insufficiently padded peripheral venous access.

Summary and Recommendations

This case reminds us that the anaesthetist should act as advocate for the patient. Not only the anaesthesia but the whole perioperative process should be kept under the anaesthetist's watchful eye.

Surgery can cause a moderate increase in CK; however, the increase should be minimal after minor surgery in children.

Careful padding of the hub of venous cannulas, as well as ensuring that the attachment of the pulse oximeter sensor is not too tight, can avoid damage.

References

Bocca, G., van Moorselaar, J.A., Feitz, W.F., et al. (2002). Compartment syndrome, rhabdomyolysis and risk of acute renal failure as complications of the lithotomy position. *J Nephrol*, 15, 183–185.

Ceran, C., Taner, O.F., Tekin, F., et al. (2012). Management of pulse oximeter probe-induced finger injuries in children: report of two consecutive cases and review of the literature. *J Pediatr Surg*, 47, e27–e29.

Laurence, A.S. (2000). Serum myoglobin and creatine kinase following surgery. *Br J Anaesth*, 84, 763–766.

Mouzopoulos, G., Kouvaris, C., Antonopoulos, D., et al. (2007). Perioperative creatine phosphokinase (CPK) and troponin I trends after elective hip surgery. *J Trauma*, 63, 388–393.

Poli, D., Gemma, M., Cozzi, S., et al. (2007). Muscle enzyme elevation after elective neurosurgery. *Eur J Anaesthesiol*, 24, 551–555.

Srinivasan, C. & Kuppuswamy, B. (2012). Rhabdomyolysis complicating non-invasive blood pressure measurement. *Indian J Anaesth*, 56, 428–430.

Swei, S.C., Liou, C.C., Liu, H.H., et al. (2009). Acute radial nerve injury associated with an automatic blood pressure monitor. *Acta Anaesthesiol Taiwan*, 47, 147–149.

Yousef, M.A., Vaida, S., Somri, M., et al. (2006). Changes in creatine phosphokinase (CK) concentrations after minor and major surgeries in children. *Br J Anaesth*, 96, 786–789.

Case 8.2

Damage Caused by Positioning

Case

Decades ago, a 16-year-old girl, weighing 72 kg, was scheduled for Nuss repair of pectus excavatum. After intravenous sedation a thoracic epidural catheter was inserted via an 18G Tuohy needle at the T6/T7 level and loaded with 8 ml bupivacaine 0.25% including 0.5 mg morphine. Anaesthesia was induced with propofol, fentanyl and mivacurium. The airway was secured with a 37F double-lumen tube and the correct position was confirmed by fibreoptic inspection. For maintenance, desflurane and a mivacurium infusion were used.

The patient was positioned with both arms abducted 90°, at the request of the surgeon. It was a re-do procedure, and surgery was demanding. The surgeon claimed that he was constrained by an insufficiently abducted arm, and he moved it more towards the head of the patient, despite the anaesthetist's comment that this could endanger the brachial plexus.

During the case bupivacaine 0.25% was infused at a rate of 4 ml/h over the epidural catheter; in addition, before extubation, a bolus of 4 ml bupivacaine 0.75% was given. Postoperatively patient-controlled epidural analgesia with bupivacaine 0.125% plus fentanyl 2 μg/ml was used. Therefore, initially weakness of the right arm was attributed to the analgesia technique; however, weakness persisted after reduction and then cessation of the local anaesthetic administration. The diagnosis of brachial plexus palsy was confirmed. There was some improvement over the next few weeks, but even after 3 months the patient was still relevantly impaired during her daily activities.

Discussion

This case of injury to the **brachial plexus** due to abduction of the arm by over 90° at the shoulder illustrates that positioning can cause nerve damage in children too. They are not resistant to this type of injury. In adults brachial plexus injury is the second most common nerve injury associated with anaesthesia (Cheney et al. 1999). During the Nuss procedure the surgeon needs access to the lateral chest wall, and abduction of the arms is usually requested; however, with abduction of over 90° a 5.1% incidence of transient brachial plexus injury has been reported in this type of surgery (Fox et al. 2005). During cardiac catheterization the arms are often placed hyperextended behind the head, with the risk of over-stretching the brachial plexus (Souza Neto et al. 1998). However, such a position is routinely used for diagnostic imaging, e.g. for CT scans, with no negative sequelae; therefore the duration of ischaemia seems to be critical. Rotation of the head towards the abducted arm seems to alleviate the stress on the brachial plexus.

The **ulnar nerve** can be exposed to direct pressure at the elbow and is the most commonly injured nerve during anaesthesia (Cheney et al. 1999). The elbow should be

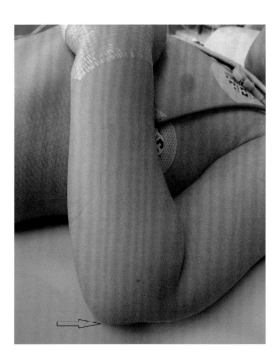

Figure 8.2 Positioning the arm with the elbow flexed 90° has a high risk for ulnar nerve damage. This undesirable position has to be avoided when children are placed in the lithotomy position.

extended and well padded, with the arm preferably in a supinated position (Prielipp *et al.* 1999). The author has personally encountered an ulnar nerve injury in a schoolchild whose arm was positioned with the elbow flexed 90° on the operating table (Fig. 8.2).

In the lower extremity, the **peroneal nerve** is extremely sensitive to pressure, and especially in the lateral position meticulous care is needed to provide sufficient padding of the region around the fibular head. The author once came across a 4-year-old child who had a foot drop for several weeks after renal surgery in the lateral position. Peroneal nerve palsy can also occur after the use of extension devices on a fracture table for femoral fractures in children (Kelly *et al.* 2017); often the non-operated side, which is less well under control during surgery, is affected. Even in a supine patient, an extreme knee-out position can put the peroneal nerve at risk, especially when the operation takes place in the genital region and the legs are covered by the surgical drapes.

Beside nerve injuries from stretching or direct pressure, **pressure sores and skin necrosis** can also occur. In very prolonged cases, e.g. over 4 hours, even perfect padding does not exclude every risk, and it is a good practice occasionally to move the patient's head and if possible the heels just a few millimetres, in order to change the pressure that the tissues are exposed to.

In very delicate patients, normally well-tolerated manoeuvres can lead to **fractures**. The author remembers more than one femoral fracture caused by positioning and rotations of the leg for heel lancing in preterm babies. And of course the child with osteogenesis imperfecta is a special challenge for the paediatric anaesthetist.

The **Nuss procedure** is a minimally invasive repair of pectus excavatum which was developed by Nuss in 1987 and has in many places replaced the traditional Ravitch technique. Although the perioperative course is in most cases uneventful, the technique carries several risks which are of concern for the anaesthetist: he or she has to be prepared for dysrhythmias, vascular injury, cardiac perforation, pneumothorax, pleural effusion and haemorrhage. Over almost 20 years the author has personally encountered life-threatening arrhythmias, pneumothorax and pleural effusions, in addition to the brachial plexus palsy of the case described.

Perioperative medicine is a 'team sport'. High performance by all team members is needed for a good outcome. This is well illustrated by the topic of positioning. The surgeon requires good access to the surgical field, whereas for the anaesthetist minimal interference with ventilation and emergency access to the airway and the intravascular catheters are primary concerns. Both are responsible for ensuring that everything is in the best interest of the patient and that no damage occurs. In some countries the legal aspects of this collaboration are discussed in detail (Auerhammer 2008). In paediatric patients, positioning can interfere extensively with the function of the devices of the anaesthetist as well as with access to the patient, and therefore correct positioning should be among the core competencies of the paediatric anaesthetist.

Summary and Recommendations

This case of brachial plexus palsy illustrates that the whole perioperative team should pay attention that the arms are not unnecessarily abducted more than 90°.

The ulnar and the peroneal nerve are extremely sensitive to pressure.

Even with correct padding, pressure sores or even skin necrosis can occur, and minimal position changes now and then are recommended.

References

Auerhammer, J. (2008). Positioning of the patient for surgery [in German]. *Anaesthesist*, 57, 1107–1124.

Cheney, F.W., Domino, K.B., Caplan, R.A., *et al.* (1999). Nerve injury associated with anesthesia: a closed claims analysis. *Anesthesiology*, 90, 1062–1069.

Fox, M.E., Bensard, D.D., Roaten, J.B., *et al.* (2005). Positioning for the Nuss procedure: avoiding brachial plexus injury. *Paediatr Anaesth*, 15, 1067–1071.

Kelly, B.A., Naqvi, M., Rademacher, E.S., *et al.* (2017). Fracture table application for pediatric femur fractures: incidence and risk factors associated with adverse outcomes. *J Pediatr Orthop*, 37, e353–e356.

Prielipp, R.C., Morell, R.C., Walker, F.O., *et al.* (1999). Ulnar nerve pressure: influence of arm position and relationship to somatosensory evoked potentials. *Anesthesiology*, 91, 345–354.

Souza Neto, E.P., Durand, P.G., Sassolas, F., *et al.* (1998). Brachial plexus injury during cardiac catheterisation in children: report of two cases. *Acta Anaesthesiol Scand*, 42, 876–879.

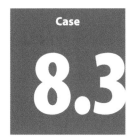

Case 8.3

Iatrogenic Burns

Case

Many decades ago, a 2-day-old neonate, 3.5 kg, was scheduled for emergency laparotomy because of suspected intestinal obstruction. Following intravenous induction with 4 mg/kg thiopental and 0.2 mg/kg pancuronium, anaesthesia was maintained with isoflurane in air and oxygen.

The right radial artery was successfully cannulated at the second attempt, using the transillumination technique with 'cold light' borrowed from the surgical team. The 2F arterial catheter (Seldicath Plastimed) was sutured in place and a bandage with a dorsal splint was applied. On the dorsum of the wrist a 4 mm diameter white skin area was seen, but it was thought to be irrelevant. But 2 days later the paediatric surgeon drew the anaesthetist's attention to a 'mysterious' necrotic skin area on the dorsum of the baby's wrist (Fig. 8.3). After excision and primary surgical closure the further course was uneventful, as no damage to the underlying tendons had occurred.

Discussion

This case of an **iatrogenic burn** caused by a **'cold light'** source dramatically illustrates that this device is not cold at all (Hindle *et al.* 2009). Numerous other cases of burns have been reported when such 'cold light' sources were used for transillumination for vascular access (Sümpelmann *et al.* 2006) or diagnosis of a pneumothorax (Sajben *et al.* 1999). At first glance, as in this case, the origin of the skin lesions may not be obvious to colleagues not directly involved in the procedure (Sajben *et al.* 1999). Following this case, the author first packed some ice-cubes into the sterile glove used for covering the light source, but then started to use pocket lamps. **Pocket lamps** generated less heat, but were still hot enough to cause blister formation. Today, only **LED devices** can be recommended.

The majority of iatrogenic burns are probably associated with the **surgical procedure**. The author remembers the smoke caused by the ignition of the surgical drape followed by a third-degree burn mark at the décolleté neckline of a young girl when the fibreoptic light source was directed onto the thorax at the termination of a cystoscopy. Perioperative medicine is a 'team sport'; therefore the anaesthetist has to react immediately when he or she spots such a situation.

The risk of burns caused by **electric current** also has to be considered. During the use of monopolar cautery, an insufficiently adherent negative plate can induce severe burns. Similarly, during an MRI examination, the rapidly changing magnetic field induces a current in ECG leads forming a loop. This is then responsible for skin burns.

The risk of burning the skin is relatively low with today's **forced-air warming devices**. However, the skin should not come into direct contact with the air hose connection, and the

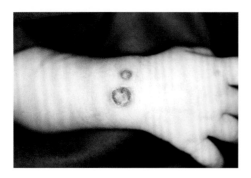

Figure 8.3 Skin burn caused by a surgical cold light during radial arterial cannulation.

circulating air flow in the mattress should not be obstructed (Azzam & Krock 1995, Stewart & Harban 2012). A towel should be placed between the air hose connection and the adjacent leg or arm. Electric heating pads, not designed for medical use, must not be used during anaesthesia and intensive care. When these have become extensively soaked by body fluids, even lethal burns have been observed.

There is always an increased **risk of fire** (Rinder 2008) when oxygen is flooding the surgical field, inflammable substances are present (Culp *et al.* 2013), e.g. not yet fully dried alcoholic skin disinfection (Bonnet *et al.* 2015), and when ignition is enhanced, e.g. by cautery or laser application. When surgery using cautery or laser is performed in the head or neck region, nasal oxygen administration should be avoided during monitored anaesthesia care, and the oxygen concentration should be set as low as justifiable during general anaesthesia. Most surgical fires happen because the people involved do not think about this possibility. In the past, when ether and cyclopropane were everywhere in use, the risk of fires and explosions was always present in the mind of the anaesthetist (Macdonald 1994a, 1994b). We should not forget the lessons learned from the past.

In addition, the author has seen countless cases of skin burns or scalds caused by medical heat application or the spillage of hot water used for inhalation for upper respiratory tract infections.

Summary and Recommendations

So-called 'cold light' must not come into contact with the patient's skin because of the high risk of burn injuries. For transillumination only LED devices should be used.

Forced-air warming devices can cause burns when the air hose connection comes into direct contact with the skin.

When there is an increased risk of ignition and fire, the oxygen concentration must be set as low as possible.

References

Azzam, F.J. & Krock, J.L. (1995). Thermal burns in two infants associated with a forced air warming system. *Anesth Analg*, 81, 661.

Bonnet, A., Devienne, M., De Brouker, V., *et al.* (2015). Operating room fire: should we mistrust alcoholic antiseptics? *Ann Chir Plast Esthet*, 60, 255–261.

Culp, W.C., Kimbrough, B.A., & Luna, S. (2013). Flammability of surgical drapes and materials in varying concentrations of oxygen. *Anesthesiology*, 119, 770–776.

Hindle, A.K., Brody, F., Hopkins, V., *et al.* (2009). Thermal injury secondary to laparoscopic fiber-optic cables. *Surg Endosc*, 23, 1720–1723.

Macdonald, A.G. (1994a). A brief historical review of non-anaesthetic causes of fires and explosions in the operating room. *Br J Anaesth*, 73, 847–856.

Macdonald, A.G. (1994b). A short history of fires and explosions caused by anaesthetic agents. *Br J Anaesth*, 72, 710–722.

Rinder, C.S. (2008). Fire safety in the operating room. *Curr Opin Anaesthesiol*, 21, 790–795.

Sajben, F.P., Gibbs, N.F., & Friedlander, S.F. (1999). Transillumination blisters in a neonate. *J Am Acad Dermatol*, 41, 264–265.

Stewart, C. & Harban, F. (2012). Thermal injuries from the use of a forced-air warming device. *Paediatr Anaesth*, 22, 414–415.

Sümpelmann, R., Osthaus, W.A., Irmler, H., *et al.* (2006). Prevention of burns caused by transillumination for peripheral venous access in neonates. *Paediatr Anaesth*, 16, 1097–1098.

Toxic Skin Necrosis

Case

Decades ago, a 6-year-old girl, 20 kg, was scheduled for major urological surgery. Anaesthesia was induced intravenously with thiopental, fentanyl and mivacurium. The airway was secured with a size 5.0 cuffed endotracheal tube (ETT) which was well lubricated and passed easily through the nostril into the trachea. The nose and the cheek were cleaned with petroleum ether to degrease the skin and the tube was taped in place. Following institutional practice, a suture was knotted around the tube to guarantee good bonding of the tape on the tube.

Anaesthesia was maintained with desflurane and a mivacurium infusion, and a caudal block containing morphine 50 µg/kg was performed for postoperative analgesia. The anaesthetic course was uneventful, and after more than 6 hours the girl was extubated. The residual adhesive was removed from the skin, again using petroleum ether. The skin which had been covered by the tapes appeared moist but not severely damaged; 2 days later, however, superficial skin necrosis was evident (Fig. 8.4a). The area was covered with ointment and healed; however, several years later, scarring of the skin at the tip of the nose was still visible.

Discussion

This case of **toxic skin necrosis** caused by petroleum ether ultimately triggered the permanent ban of this compound from the author's working environment. **Petroleum ether** (called *Wundbenzin* in German) is not an ether in the chemical sense, but a mixture of saturated hydrocarbons, e.g. pentane, hexane, heptane. It is widely used in the medical field and present in many households to remove residual glue from tapes and to clean the skin. In contrast to ethanol and isopropanol, it is not suitable for skin disinfection. Basically, the compound is toxic, both systemically and locally (Parasuraman *et al.* 2014). When it is applied to the skin for cleaning and allowed to evaporate for a sufficient time, it may be used uneventfully. But when it is covered by an occlusive dressing, in this case by the tapes used for tube fixation, the highly lipophilic agent penetrates deeply into the skin and causes skin necrosis, which is typically only fully visible with a latency of 1 day. In this case the tight suture around the tube perhaps increased the mechanical stress to the skin at the tip of the patient's nose.

The author has been responsible for three **additional cases** of skin toxicity by petroleum ether. A patient developed a deep black skin necrosis on the forehead following the placement of an ECG electrode after removal of makeup with petroleum ether. A preterm baby developed deep skin necrosis needing repeated surgery after the fixation of an intravenous line in the great saphenous vein with a Tegaderm; in this patient, the senior nurse had commented that the use of ethyl ether would be safer. Finally, a 4-year-old child developed a palm-sized toxic skin reaction over the sacral region after the removal of landmarks drawn for teaching a caudal block; in this case no occlusive dressing was used, but a large amount of petroleum ether was rubbed forcefully over the skin and thereafter the child was predominantly in the supine position (Fig. 8.4b). Although experienced nurses often know of this toxic phenomenon, surprisingly, it is not mentioned in the medical literature. And it took more than half of his professional life for the author to realize the relevance of this issue.

What are the **alternatives** for degreasing the skin and increasing the adhesion of the tape? **Ethyl ether** effectively removes residual glue and rapidly evaporates; some seconds later the tape can be applied without negative consequences. The disadvantages are the distinctive smell and the risk of forming an explosive mixture with oxygen (Macdonald 1994). Especially when it is used for fixation of the ETT, in case of a leaky tube, high concentrations of oxygen may be present around the area of application. Nevertheless, with appropriate care, ethyl ether was successfully used over many years in the author's institution. Commercially available solutions, e.g. Cavilon, provide a rapidly drying protective skin film followed by good adherence of the tape. For the removal of residual glue, Niltac, a silicon-based rapidly evaporating fluid, can be used.

Solutions used for **skin disinfection**, especially alcohol-based solutions, can cause large-scale skin damage when applied in excess and left undried for a prolonged time. The author

(a)

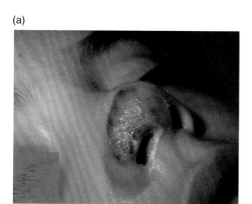

Figure 8.4a Toxic skin damage after cleaning the skin with petroleum ether followed by firmly taping the ETT in place.

(b)

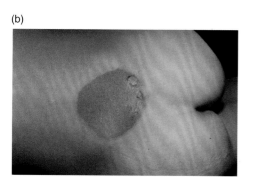

Figure 8.4b Toxic skin damage after cleaning the skin with petroleum ether to remove landmarks that were drawn for teaching caudal block.

remembers a 10-year-old boy who suffered severe skin necrosis on the scrotum after a femoral nerve block and insufficient removal of the alcoholic povidone solution. After any invasive intervention in the groin, the skin between thigh and scrotum or labia majora has to be carefully cleaned and dried.

Summary and Recommendations

This case shows that we should ban petroleum ether (*Wundbenzin* in German) from the anaesthetic environment, because when it is covered by tapes severe skin toxicity can occur.

After performing invasive procedures, residual disinfection solution has to be removed and the skin carefully dried, especially in intertriginous body regions.

This series of skin necrosis caused by petroleum ether shows that individual and institutional learning can be very slow.

References

Macdonald, A.G. (1994). A short history of fires and explosions caused by anaesthetic agents. *Br J Anaesth*, 72, 710–722.

Parasuraman, S., Sujithra, J., Syamittra, B., *et al.* (2014). Evaluation of sub-chronic toxic effects of petroleum ether, a laboratory solvent in Sprague-Dawley rats. *J Basic Clin Pharm*, 5, 89–97.

Case

Decades ago, a 10-year-old boy, weighing 28 kg, was brought to the hospital by ambulance after a traffic accident. He had suffered an open leg fracture and extensive skin avulsion. After the initial survey, blood sampling and x-ray examination he was brought to the OR for external fixation and wound debridement under general endotracheal anaesthesia. Over the next 3 days he underwent daily wound revisions under general anaesthesia. Each time, because of profuse bleeding, one or two units of packed red cells were needed to keep the haemoglobin at 80 g/l. A slight jaundice and the unexpectedly high need for transfusions initiated further investigations. In addition, according to the local guidelines, after 96 hours type and screen had to be repeated.

It was only now, when type and screen was repeated, that the haematology laboratory reported that the patient's real blood group did not correspond to the blood group found in the tubes initially sampled in the emergency room. It was clear that blood tubes had been mixed up during this process. Surprisingly, it was not possible to uncover the details of this error.

Discussion

This case of a **haemolytic transfusion reaction** caused by a mix-up of blood samples during the process of blood sampling and labelling makes the point that every time blood is taken from a patient and labelled with the patient's name this is a matter of life and death. 'Wrong blood in tube' has to be avoided (Ansari & Szallasi 2011). Labelling the tubes containing freshly sampled blood is probably the most error-prone step in the process, especially because, at that moment, several people are likely to be involved. Most severe haemolytic reactions probably result from human error (Stainsby *et al.* 2008). Happily, in this patient, only a delayed haemolytic reaction occurred. Acute intravascular haemolysis would have been immediately life-threatening; it leads to shock, coagulopathy, renal damage and hyperkalaemia. Following this case, similar to the procedure in other institutions (Ansari & Szallasi 2011), the institutional practice was changed: every previously un-typed recipient of blood now needs a second determination of blood group in addition to the first 'type and screen' test, and in every unit of blood leaving the haematology laboratory the blood group is determined once more, although, of course, it is labelled with the blood group and has undergone extensive testing beforehand.

In addition, many other **hazards of blood transfusions** exist (Harrison & Bolton 2011). Everybody is talking about the infectious risks, but with modern testing the risk of acquiring **viral diseases** is extremely low. On the other hand, **bacterial contamination** is

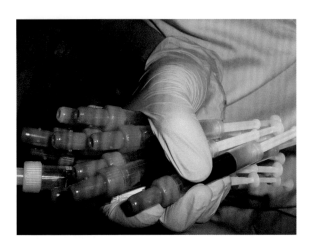

Figure 8.5 Blood taken from a preschool child for further investigations. Minimizing iatrogenic losses by repeated blood sampling can reduce the transfusion frequency.

still a problem and associated with a high mortality. Notably, this risk in addition to the risk of confusions is not excluded by preoperative autologous donation. But in any case, preoperative autologous donation has been abandoned almost completely for various reasons: stored autologous blood seems to have a negative immunological impact similar to that of donated blood; in addition, a lower haematocrit before surgery will increase the likelihood of a transfusion during surgery, and cost and especially the logistic and emotional efforts in paediatric patients are not negligible.

Most transfusion reactions are **febrile or allergic non-haemolytic reactions**. However, the uniform use of leucodepletion has made them much less common. The most dangerous blood products in use are platelet concentrates. In the author's experience, transfusion-related **circulatory overload** was the most common complication, especially at the beginning of his career. He remembers a child with tonsillar re-bleeding who presented, although actively bleeding, with severe anaemia with haemoglobin of 50 g/l. The rapid administration of two units of blood induced a fulminant pulmonary oedema. In clinical practice, distinguishing between acute and predominantly chronic bleeding can be challenging.

Avoiding transfusions completely is the optimal way to avoid a transfusion reaction. The concept in vogue of **patient blood management** has reached paediatric anaesthesia too (Cholette *et al.* 2017). Realistically, only rarely can preoperative anaemia be corrected with acceptable effort. But adherence to transfusion guidelines (Kozek-Langenecker *et al.* 2017), the use of tranexamic acid and especially minimizing iatrogenic losses by repeated large-volume blood sampling (Steffen *et al.* 2017) are important steps to be considered (Fig. 8.5).

Summary and Recommendations

This case illustrates that 'wrong blood in tube' is a continuously present threat; every effort is needed to avoid it.

Minimizing the blood volume taken at phlebotomy should be one target of future technical developments.

References

Ansari, S. & Szallasi, A. (2011). 'Wrong blood in tube': solutions for a persistent problem. *Vox Sang*, 100, 298–302.

Cholette, J.M., Faraoni, D., Goobie, S.M., *et al.* (2017). Patient blood management in pediatric cardiac surgery: a review. *Anesth Analg*, 5 October, doi: 10.1213/ ANE.0000000000002504 [ePub ahead of print].

Harrison, E. & Bolton, P. (2011). Serious hazards of transfusion in children (SHOT). *Paediatr Anaesth*, 21, 10–13.

Kozek-Langenecker, S.A., Ahmed, A.B., Afshari, A., *et al.* (2017). Management of severe perioperative bleeding: guidelines from the European Society of Anaesthesiology: first update 2016. *Eur J Anaesthesiol*, 34, 332–395.

Stainsby, D., Jones, H., Wells, A.W., *et al.* (2008). Adverse outcomes of blood transfusion in children: analysis of UK reports to the serious hazards of transfusion scheme 1996–2005. *Br J Haematol*, 141, 73–79.

Steffen, K., Doctor, A., Hoerr, J., *et al.* (2017). Controlling phlebotomy volume diminishes PICU transfusion: implementation processes and impact. *Pediatrics*, 140, pii: e20162480.

Index